ROTTENSEED!
Cottonseed, Alzheimer's and Your Brain

BY

BRUCE SEMON, MD, PhD.

Wisconsin Institute of Nutrition, LLP
Milwaukee, Wisconsin
www.nutritioninstitute.com

Disclaimer

Rottenseed! Cottonseed, Alzheimer's and Your Brain describes relationships which have been observed between cottonseed in food and various health conditions. The sole intention of this book is to provide information, not provide medical treatment. This book is not intended to substitute for the judgment of your health care provider. The publisher and its authors are not liable for any misuse or misunderstanding of the information contained in this book. If any reader has particular health questions, please see your health care provider. This book is not a prescription for health or wellness. Neither the author nor Wisconsin Institute of Nutrition, LLP, has any liability or responsibility to any person or entity with respect to any loss, damage or injury caused or alleged to be caused by the information contained in this book.

ROTTENSEED! Cottonseed, Alzheimer's and Your Brain
Wisconsin Institute of Nutrition, LLP
http://www.nutritioninstitute.com; 877-332-7899

Library of Congress Catalog in Publication Data
Semon, Bruce, M.D., Ph.D.,
Rottenseed! Cottonseed, Alzheimer's and Your Brain

Includes Index
1. Alzheimer's
2. Alzheimer's Disease
3. Cottonseed
4. Atherosclerosis
5. Stroke
6. Gossypol
7. Cyclopropenoid fatty acids
8. Benzo(a)pyrene

ISBN: 0-9670057-2-8
ISBN 13: 9780967005720
Library of Congress Control Number: 2013941305
Wisconsin Institute of Nutrition,
Milwaukee WI

This book is dedicated to my wife,
Lori Kornblum,
and our children,
AVRAHAM, SARAH AND MIKAH

ABOUT THE AUTHOR

Bruce Semon, M.D., Ph.D., is a board certified psychiatrist in both Child and Adolescent and Adult psychiatry. He holds a Ph.D. in Nutrition from University of California, Davis. He received his medical degree (M.D.) from University of Wisconsin, Madison, and did further research work at National Institutes of Health, National Cancer Institute in Maryland. He received his certifications in Adult and Child and Adolescent Psychiatry from Medical College of Wisconsin. Dr. Semon has published numerous academic papers in peer-reviewed journals. Dr. Semon has a particular interest in how what people eat affect their health. He has lectured nationally and internationally on how changing diet affects health.

Dr. Semon is also the author of......

- ✓ *Feast Without Yeast: 4 Stages to Better Health,* by Bruce Semon, M.D., Ph.D., and Lori Kornblum (Wisconsin Institute of Nutrition, LLP, 1999), explains Dr. Semon's yeast free, gluten free and dairy free dietary approach to treating common problems caused by the yeast Candida albicans, including autism, ADHD, multiple sclerosis, chronic fatigue syndrome, fibromyalgia, ulcerative colitis, Crohn's Disease, Tourette's Syndrome, and other problems. Feast Without Yeast also contains more than 225 recipes, and is now a standard in the field of cooking for special diets.

- ✓ An *Extraordinary Power to Heal*, by Bruce Semon, M.D., Ph.D., and Lori Kornblum (Wisconsin Institute of Nutrition, LLP, 2003) explains the scientific basis for how *Candida albicans* causes many major and significant health problems.

✓ ***Extraordinary Foods for the Everyday Kitchen***, by Bruce Semon, M.D., Ph.D., and Lori Kornblum (Wisconsin Institute of Nutrition, LLP, 2003) is a yeast free, gluten free and dairy free cookbook filled with delicious and outstanding recipes and menus.

✓ ***Biological Treatments for Autism and P.D.D.***, by Dr. William Shaw, contributing author

TABLE OF CONTENTS

FOREWORD

I am writing this book to help people understand the tremendous risk to health coming from cottonseed toxins in our food. When I was at the National Cancer Institute in 1989, I was studying lists of cancer causing chemicals in our food. On some of those lists were the cottonseed toxins because they cause genetic mutations. I thought it very strange at the time that cottonseed was part of our food. I did not know much about cottonseed when I began studying the agricultural feeding practice of feeding cottonseed to animals. Cottonseed is fed heavily to animals, to cattle, to chickens, to farm fed fish, and to pigs. But cottonseed contains poisons. One of these poisons, gossypol, goes to the brain and literally ties important structures together. I thought it was an ideal candidate for causing Alzheimer's. The problem was that I could not interest anyone in the National Cancer Institute or in the National Institute on Aging that this was an idea worth testing. I left the National Cancer Institute after doing other work for two years and decided that someday I would test this idea about gossypol myself. Finally in 2004, I put together an animal lab and fed rats for three years small amounts of cottonseed every day to see if they would develop Alzheimer's. This book is about the thinking that went into this experiment, the results and the implications for the food we all consume and the health of everyone.

I want to thank Mr. Carsten Wordell for his expert help with animal care. I want to thank Dr. Dan Schenkman for his expert help with animal pathology. I want to thank Sarah Semon for her help with animal care and with editing this book. I want to thank my dear wife Lori Kornblum for her tremendous help in editing this book. I want to think Dr. Shmuel Mandelbaum for taking the cover photograph of the author.

CHAPTER 1

ROTTENSEED! COTTONSEED, ALZHEIMER'S AND YOU: AN INTRODUCTION THAT COULD SAVE YOUR LIFE

This book is about Alzheimer's, heart disease, and you. This book is about avoiding these problems in your life by not eating one highly poisonous item: cottonseed.

Cottonseed?

Yes.

Cottonseed contains toxic chemicals.

Although cottonseed is not really a food, and although you don't eat it like you eat sunflower seeds or pumpkin seeds, cottonseed is used as an animal food and as cooking oil and has saturated our food supply. It is present directly in almost every processed food, and it is present indirectly in much of our meat, dairy, poultry and fish.

Why have you not heard about this before? The answer is simple. Until now, the question of what are the health effects of cottonseed has rarely been researched and even when researched, has not been publicized. This book changes all that. I will tell you in this book that agricultural scientists began researching more than a century ago exactly how to feed cottonseed to animals without killing them. They researched this question to help cotton farmers figure out what to do with a major waste problem from cotton production: the seeds of the cotton plants. What better way to get rid of a waste byproduct than to feed it to animals and make it into human food? Scientists had to research the question of how much cottonseed could be fed to animals because unlimited cottonseed feeding killed the animals which ate the cottonseed.

But with few exceptions, scientists have not asked whether feeding the extremely toxic cottonseed to animals over their lifetimes, and whether putting cottonseed oil directly in food, has an impact on human health. Nor have scientists asked the question whether people can safely eat cottonseed over the course of their lifetimes. Why not? In a later chapter, we will see that these scientists had no incentive to ask such questions.

However, as you will see later, cottonseed toxins may be very important in Alzheimer's. This information is not much known publicly. But as of today from the perspective of the general public, Alzheimer's is devastating to patients and their families. With all of the billions spent on health care in this country, people might think that doctors and scientists should know how to reduce the risk of Alzheimer's. Why can't these medical scientists figure out how to prevent this illness? Maybe for these medical scientists, information is missing or is unavailable or is too complex or is politically out of bounds. Perhaps scientists are asking the wrong questions or have missed some important relevant information.

I raised this question about Alzheimer's and cottonseed toxins. As a Ph.D. in nutrition, as well as board certified medical doctor, I am interested in looking at how people may be able to prevent disease by changing what they eat. This book is about prevention, not treatment. This book is not about the drugs that are currently prescribed for Alzheimer's symptoms. I am familiar with these drugs. They slow down but do not cure the disease. In my view, based on my contact with Alzheimer's patients, one should try to prevent the illness because once it takes hold on the brain, it is devastating.

I had to fund the research privately. I performed the experiments. The results were remarkable, and have been published in a peer reviewed journal.[1] As I explain in this book, the road to doing all this was not easy. I have found that feeding cottonseed toxins to rats caused Alzheimer's as well as many other health problems.

You may be skeptical. After all, if cottonseed is ubiquitous in our food supply, it must be safe. Surely government agencies will protect us. I will show you why that assumption of safety is wrong. I will show you that cottonseed toxins in amounts comparable to those that the average consumer eats caused Alzheimer's, heart disease and other major health problems in rats.

You may also be skeptical because you think this is another passing fad. Every day, Americans are besieged with information about why this, that or the other thing is bad for them. The information becomes so confusing that many people just give up.

The information I present here is based on science. I am not selling anything. Many of the agencies and people who want you to change your habits are selling supplements, drugs or exercise equipment to help you. Unfortunately, there is no supplement or drug to counteract cottonseed toxins. I am only presenting information.

What is cottonseed?

Ironically, reducing the risk of Alzheimer's starts by understanding a plant that mainly ends up in clothing: cotton. Cotton is a plant that grows in many areas in the United States. The white, fluffy fibers of cotton are woven into cloth that has a lovely texture and feels great against the skin.

These plant fibers are attached to large seeds. In nature, the seeds hold onto the fibers for dispersal, similar to the way dandelion fibers hold onto dandelion seeds for dispersal when people blow on them. The seeds in cotton, however, are not tiny like dandelion seeds, but very large, brown and hard.

Until the early 1800's, separating the cotton fibers from the seeds was extremely time consuming. Cotton cloth could not be mass-produced because this separation was too labor intensive. In 1793, Eli Whitney invented the cotton gin, which solved this problem. The cotton gin allowed for mechanical separation of the cotton fibers from the seeds. Although the cotton gin has been refined since 1793, it is still a mechanical separator.

The cotton gin allowed for mass production of cotton fiber. However, the solution to one problem led to another: large amounts of cottonseed waste.

According to the website of the National Cottonseed Products Association,[2] initially cottonseed was plowed back into the ground or left to rot in heaps. After the Civil War, however, farmers began to use cottonseed as animal feed because, like all seeds, the cotton seeds contain protein necessary to support new plant life. The National Cottonseed Products Association continues. "Cottonseed feed products have been used for the feeding of livestock for more than 150 years." More than 20 million tons of cottonseed is produced around the world and is fed to animals. Cottonseed is used in many ways:

"Cottonseed Meal, Cottonseed Hulls and Whole Cottonseed are natural sources of protein, fiber and energy. Cottonseed meal is the most abundant plant protein feed available throughout the U.S., after soybean meal. It can be used in both ruminant (cows with several stomachs) and monogastric (one stomach such as in pigs) rations. Cottonseed hulls are a valuable source of roughage for ruminant feeds and fiber for monogastric rations. Whole and delinted cottonseed are concentrated sources of protein and energy for ruminant rations."[3]

What the cottonseed producers don't mention is that feeding cottonseed to animals causes problems. In post Civil War times, many farm animals died from eating cottonseed. Dead animals caused problems for the farmers! The problem was termed "cottonseed injury," and was recognized back in the 1800's after the Civil War, soon after farmers began using cottonseed as animal feed. In early years, this problem was noted in horses, cattle and sheep, but especially in pigs. Cottonseed injury resulted in the animals' lungs filling with fluid, like pneumonia. Their hearts would fail and they would bleed to death. In a 1915 paper on cottonseed, the authors wrote that" cottonseed was being fed 'profitably' to horses, cattle, and sheep but only if they became accustomed to the cottonseed." Farmers could not feed pigs cottonseed at that time because it was too toxic for them. The authors of this 1915 paper comment: "While it may be fed profitably to horses, cattle and sheep, etc., in moderate amounts, poisoning and often death occur as a result, especially if the animal has not been gradually accustomed to it. It is generally avoided as a feed for pigs on account of the numerous deaths associated with its use."[4]

Since 1915, agricultural researchers have devoted much time and effort to figuring out how safely to feed cottonseed to farm animals so that they do not become ill or die. Researchers tried to detoxify the cottonseed and separate out the poisons from the cottonseed, but had very limited success. They mainly determined how to limit the amount of cottonseed fed to animals so that the animals lived rather than died. This research enabled farmers to feed cottonseed to cattle, farm fed fish, pigs and poultry without all the risks that were described in 1915.

But what happened to all the poisons? Did the poisons disappear after the animals ate them or remain in the meat and fat of the animals? Did those poisons pose any risk to human beings who then ate the meat of these cottonseed fed animals? The other question is: what about feeding cottonseed products directly to people? Processors discovered that cottonseed oil was profitable. This oil has been used in many processed foods. What happens to the toxins in cottonseed oil? Are the toxins still present in the oil? Are these products safe for people?

Unfortunately, as I will show you in this book, the poisons do end up and remain in the meat and fat of the animals, and are present in cottonseed oil. They potentially pose a great risk to humans. To understand answers to these questions about risk, continue reading with me.

The risk of eating cottonseed toxins

Most people are aware that eating a healthy diet is important to staying healthy. Many people know that dietary choices may affect health and risk of disease. For example, people have been told that eating a high fat diet is bad for their hearts and is a risk to their health. They may choose to eat such a diet anyway because they are willing to take the risk.

People take risks all the time. Every person who drives a car takes the risk of a serious accident. The risk may be very low but is nonetheless present. There are risks from chemicals in food. For some of these chemicals our government has decided how much risk is acceptable. For example, some artificial sweeteners at high levels cause cancer in animals. Yet many people want something sweet without the calories or sugar. The government has decided that the risk from small amounts of artificial sweeteners is acceptable. In this case people can choose to take the risk because the risk is out in the open.

So, to eat right, people have to know how. The more information a person has, the more that person can protect himself or herself. The USDA provides basic information about nutrition and food choices. The FDA limits certain substances in food. Doctors may give other information.

In the case of cottonseed toxins, people can't assess the risk because in the past information has not been available showing that cottonseed is toxic to people in the amounts people actually eat. The studies on cottonseed toxins have been directed only to farmers, and for allowing them to maximize the amount of cottonseed fed to animals. The studies have not been done, until now, to determine whether cottonseed in the human food supply is safe. In addition, the animal studies have been "acute" studies, that is, feeding high levels over short periods of time. Acute studies do not accurately reproduce how people ingest cottonseed toxins. People do not eat high levels of cottonseed toxins over a short period of time. Rather, people eat low levels of cottonseed toxins in their food throughout their lifetimes. When a toxin causes a problem acutely at a high dose, will that same toxin cause the same problem at a very low dose over a long period of time? These questions are difficult to answer. That is why I did my experiment: to find out the impact of long term eating of cottonseed toxins.

First, this book will present general information about cottonseed, and the state of existing research on cottonseed and its effects. The next section of the book will present information about my experiment. This section is divided into two chapters, a chapter about my hypotheses and a chapter about the actual experiment and the results. Next, I present information about what you can do to prevent major diseases such as Alzheimer's and why you should do this. A later chapter of the book contains my suggestions for further research based on what we already know. Finally, in the last chapter, I discuss why this research is not likely to be done in the ordinary course of medical research. I hope to do to further research. However, you will see that doing so requires challenging the basic structure of the political and economic reality of the cottonseed industry and the structure of the biomedical scientific industry.

Let us begin.

CHAPTER 2

COTTONSEED IS POISONOUS!
HERE'S HOW WE KNOW

To this point, I have stated that studies show that cottonseed is toxic, and that this information is based on prior studies. In this chapter, I will describe the research that agricultural scientists have done on cottonseed and what the implications of this research are for human health. This chapter summarizes those studies so people can understand the risk of eating cottonseed, based on demonstrated short term effects of cottonseed toxicity. In an appendix I describe these studies in greater detail. In a later chapter, I describe my research which builds on the existing scientific knowledge.

Cottonseed studies on excessive bleeding and abnormal blood clotting

Scientists have shown that cottonseed causes two different problems related to bleeding. Before discussing the specific problems, one needs to understand something about the mechanisms of blood clotting.

Blood clotting is an essential body process because blood vessels tear under normal use. In a normal body, blood clotting proteins come together to form a solid structure to plug these holes and tears. These small holes need to be patched up or excessive bleeding results. An example of abnormal blood clotting is in hemophilia, a disorder in which blood does not clot properly. Small tears in the blood vessels are not patched. Excessive bleeding goes into the joints and other tissues, causing arthritis and other joint problems.

Abnormal blood clotting means at least two different processes: the first is that the blood clotting factors came together to form a solid structure in the wrong place. For example, if a blood clot forms inside a coronary artery feeding the heart, then the heart does not receive enough blood; then the heart does not have enough oxygen and a heart attack occurs. The second is if clotting does not occur such as in a blood vessel with a hole or tear, then excessive bleeding results.

Cottonseed toxins cause both excessive bleeding, also called hemorrhage, and abnormal blood clotting.

Four studies show major internal hemorrhage (excessive bleeding) in animals fed cottonseed. In the first study done in 1915, researchers fed cottonseed to rabbits.[5] At that time, scientists did not know which part of the cottonseed was toxic. They tried feeding various parts of the cottonseed and tried purifying out what they thought was the toxic part. The rabbits all died in hours or days. When scientists looked at the internal organs of the dead animals, they found a number of problems, including evidence of major internal bleeding serious enough to cause death.

A second study was done in 1927 in which small amounts of a more pure version of the cottonseed toxin were injected into rats.[6] The rats died within hours, again with evidence of major internal bleeding. In a third study in 1948, scientists separated out the cottonseed pigment glands. These parts of the cottonseed contain the toxic chemicals. The scientists then force fed these cottonseed pigment glands to rats.[7] Force feeding is required because rats will not eat concentrated cottonseed pigment glands. Again, the rats died of both major internal bleeding and stopped hearts (their term).

In the last study in 1951, scientists fed cottonseed meal to rabbits and the rabbits died within one month. These scientists tried to save the rabbits by feeding them vitamin K, which is used to treat bleeding from liver disease, but the rabbits could not be saved. In this study, the scientists compared cottonseed toxins to dicumarol (Warfarin) as a control poison.[8] Dicumarol (used commercially as a rat poison) works by causing internal bleeding in the rats. This study found that the cottonseed meal had a comparable effect on bleeding as the dicumarol.

Cottonseed toxins also have been shown to cause blood clots to form in the wrong places. In the 1915 study of rabbits noted above, researchers also found blood clots in the rabbits' hearts. As noted earlier, the formation of blood clots in the wrong place can result in a blood clot entering the coronary arteries and causing a heart attack. This finding in 1915 is still significant because there is no other research even today showing the formation of a spontaneous blood clot in a normal heart.

To summarize, four separate studies show that cottonseed toxins cause excessive bleeding in animals, and one study shows that cottonseed toxins caused abnormal clotting in animals. These findings are very significant because they help us understand how and why cottonseed may be toxic to people as well.

People also suffer from major health problems due to abnormal bleeding and abnormal clotting. Abnormal bleeding in a hospital sets off emergency alarms to doctors that something must be done quickly. Many people have suffered or do suffer from blood clots in the legs, which unfortunately can cause pulmonary embolism, when the clot moves to the lungs and can cause death.

Abnormal blood clotting and bleeding are not the only problems that cottonseed toxins cause.

Cottonseed, high cholesterol and heart disease

Studies in animals have also shown that cottonseed toxins cause high cholesterol and atherosclerosis. Atherosclerosis is accumulation of cholesterol inside the walls of arteries which narrows the arteries. These are problems which also affect people. People know that cholesterol is bad because doctors tell them it is bad. So, the fact that cottonseed can cause high cholesterol is worth noting!

Before I tell people about the studies on cottonseed, let me briefly explain what cholesterol is and why high cholesterol is bad for people.

Cholesterol has a number of functions in the body. Cholesterol is part of cell membranes. Cholesterol is one of the components of the transporters in the blood which carries fat around the body in the blood. People synthesize, or make, cholesterol which must later be excreted. This is a natural process. People also take in cholesterol in their diet. Cholesterol goes through several steps on the way to being excreted. People should be able to excrete excess cholesterol which they synthesize or take in. But somehow this does not always occur normally. Cholesterol levels can go up at least partially because people cannot clear all the cholesterol. Unfortunately, high cholesterol can cause major health problems. Cholesterol can accumulate in the arteries in atherosclerotic plaques. Normally, arteries are wide open to carry blood. An atherosclerotic plaque is formed when there is break in the lining of the arterial wall allowing cholesterol to accumulate. This accumulation results in a bulge out into the open artery where blood should be flowing. If this bulge becomes big enough, then the artery cannot carry as much blood as it should. The artery can become close to, if not totally plugged up. People can have a heart attack if this buildup occurs in the heart coronary arteries. People can have a stroke when atherosclerotic plaques develop in the brain arteries.

Cottonseed and cholesterol

Cottonseed has a particular set of toxins called cyclopropenoid fatty acids, which are found in cottonseed oil after processing. Scientists studying these toxins have observed that cyclopropenoid fatty acids increase cholesterol levels in mammals and birds.

The first study published on this subject in 1959, tested various vegetable oils to see their effects on cholesterol levels in the blood. Vegetable oils, especially those with poly-unsaturated fatty acids, almost all caused lower cholesterol levels when fed to birds. These are oils such as corn oil and soybean oil. Polyunsaturated fatty acids are found in vegetable oils, and because of their structure, are liquid at room temperature. Saturated fatty acids are solid at room temperature and are found in animal tissues such as muscle and animal fat. Scientists also tested cottonseed oil. Strangely and unexpectedly, scientists found that cottonseed oil increased cholesterol in the birds.[9] This finding was unexpected because cottonseed oil contains polyunsaturated fatty acids. Scientists thought at that time that polyunsaturated fatty acids caused lower cholesterol levels. So researchers thought there must be something else in the cottonseed oil which was causing increased cholesterol. In subsequent studies, scientists found that the cottonseed chemicals causing these problems were the cyclopropenoid fatty acids.

Other scientists found that cyclopropenoid fatty acids inhibited one of the major steps in cholesterol excretion. For cholesterol to be excreted from the body, several chemical steps must occur. Cyclopropenoid fatty acids inhibit one of the major steps in cholesterol excretion. This step is that for cholesterol to be excreted, it must be attached to an unsaturated fatty acid. Cyclopropenoid fatty acids inhibit the production of unsaturated fatty acids which can bind to cholesterol.[10] If these unsaturated fatty acids are not there, cholesterol cannot be bound in the excretion process and will then accumulate.

Other researchers looked at how the cyclopropenoid fatty acids caused increased cholesterol, atherosclerosis and heart disease. In another study, scientists found in rabbits that the cyclopropenoid fatty acids caused increased cholesterol, and caused atherosclerosis and atherosclerotic plaques in only a few weeks.[11] In a separate study, feeding cottonseed to mice also increased cholesterol levels.[12]

In summary, cyclopropenoid fatty acids make it harder for the animals to excrete cholesterol. If the animals cannot clear cholesterol, cholesterol levels will go up. When cyclopropenoid fatty acids are fed to either mice or rabbits, their cholesterol levels go up tremendously. The rabbits also develop atherosclerosis in only five weeks.

As I just explained, whole cottonseed and cottonseed oil contain chemicals called cyclopropenoid fatty acids which interfere with cholesterol excretion and increase cholesterol levels. These poisons inhibit one of the major steps which need to occur in cholesterol processing for the cholesterol to be excreted. So these poisons cause increased cholesterol levels.

Relationship between human health and the animal studies: how cottonseed increases cholesterol and heart disease

Research in animals has shown that cyclopropenoid fatty acids cause increased cholesterol and development of atherosclerotic plaques. Is there any research which helps us understand whether these toxic cyclopropenoid fatty acids have anything to do with human health? There is much research showing an association between the intake of dietary fat and increased blood cholesterol. There is research showing an association between increased blood cholesterol and the increased rate of heart attacks. Do such studies leave any room for a role for cyclopropenoid fatty acids in human heart disease.

There are no such studies on cottonseed toxins and human coronary artery disease. But I would like to point out one study which suggests that cottonseed toxins may play a role. These studies are the observation that intake of eggs does not seem to do much to human cholesterol levels.

Coronary artery disease patients with high cholesterol are advised to reduce their intake of cholesterol and saturated fat. Much of the research on risk of heart disease comes from a very large study called the Framingham Study.[13] This was a study that followed people in Framingham, Massachusetts, for many years. This study is ongoing. Through this study, researchers gained valuable information about lifestyle, diet, and health. They also took blood tests and obtained other medical information. Researchers observed that increased dietary fat was found to be associated with increased blood cholesterol and with heart attacks. This series of studies looked at who in Framingham had heart attacks and what their blood levels were of such chemicals as cholesterol. The findings in the Framingham studies were interpreted to mean that foods such as eggs, which contain cholesterol, are a cause of high cholesterol and heart problems. Based on these observations, doctors today recommend not eating too much food containing high cholesterol, such as eggs. The current recommendation is to eat a few eggs a week.

However, more recent studies show eating eggs does not affect human cholesterol levels much.[14] In this study increased egg intake was associated with a modest 1% increase in cholesterol levels. But according to current research from the Framingham studies on human heart disease, eggs should be a major offender and cause much higher cholesterol. Why this puzzle? We have to look at research on cottonseed and eggs.

Other cottonseed researchers were also interested in another problem that was not totally understood at that time, called "pink white disorder in eggs."[15] Although connected to color in eggs, the results of these studies are also totally related to cholesterol. In "pink white disorder," farmers observed that when chickens were fed cottonseed, the whites of their eggs came out pink. Research showed that cyclopropenoid fatty acids caused this discoloration. There was no way for farmers to avoid this problem. Thus, farmers ceased feeding cottonseed to chickens which lay eggs. Therefore, eggs do not contain cottonseed poisons.

Eggs are the only major source of animal fat and cholesterol which does not contain cottonseed toxins, the cyclopropenoid fatty acids. They also do not cause major increases in cholesterol. Cottonseed is fed to dairy and beef cattle, chicken, pigs and farm fed fish. These food sources are all associated with increased cholesterol.

The findings on eggs suggest that increased dietary fat and cholesterol are not enough to raise cholesterol levels unless cyclopropenoid fatty acids are also present. No researcher has ever found that pure dietary fat and cholesterol without cyclopropenoid fatty acids causes increased cholesterol and heart disease. The findings on eggs suggest that cyclopropenoid fatty acids have to be present in the food for the food to cause increased cholesterol.

Male Infertility

A third problematic area for cottonseed toxins is male fertility. Researchers have known for a long time, since at least the 1940's, that cottonseed poisons interfere with male fertility. Male rats which ingested much cottonseed could not sire rat pups. [16] Based on these findings, the Chinese experimented with the cottonseed poison gossypol as a possible temporary male anti-fertility agent. A number of Chinese researchers here in the United States looked at why the cottonseed poison gossypol caused infertility in males.[17]

Researchers found that gossypol binds to microtubules and interferes with microtubule assembly in sperm.[18] Microtubules are part of the cellular structure and skeleton and are needed for sperm cells to reproduce. If microtubules cannot be assembled properly, then sperm cannot be made. The sperm counts go way down. The Chinese thought that perhaps this problem could be temporary, making gossypol a birth control agent for men. However, the result for some men taking gossypol was permanent sterility. There are no reports after this time that gossypol came into common use as a male anti-fertility agent.

However, any man wondering why his sperm count is low or why he is infertile should consider avoiding cottonseed in his diet.

The interference with microtubule assembly is also very important in development of Alzheimer's, as will be discussed shortly.

Failing hearts and fluid in lungs

In other studies of cottonseed toxicity, animals which are fed cottonseed develop failing hearts and fluid in their lungs.[19] Failing hearts and lungs filled with fluid are noted in agricultural animals such as pigs which have been fed more cottonseed than they can tolerate.

If cottonseed causes all of these problems in animals, is cottonseed safe for people? I leave readers here with the suggestion that cottonseed is not OK for people; in fact, it can be devastating. The question is, do people eat enough food containing cottonseed toxins to cause heart disease? I will come back to this question later after presenting my own research on low level cottonseed intake.

Review and summary of the research:
What does this mean for people?

Research to date shows that cottonseed toxins cause:

✓ High cholesterol

✓ Atherosclerosis and Atherosclerotic plaques

✓ Bleeding

✓ Blood Clotting

✓ Male Infertility

✓ Failing hearts

We should have another concern about cottonseed. Cottonseed contains at least 15 poisons, many of which are not well studied.[20] Gossypol and the cyclopropenoid fatty acids are some of the toxins but there are others which scientists have not studied at all. These unstudied toxins add to the toxicity of individual toxins. The toxicity of whole cottonseed (which contains all the toxins) in the diet is greater than the toxicity of gossypol in the diet alone. We don't know what these other toxins are doing but when animals receive whole cottonseed, they develop more problems than if they are fed gossypol alone.

In general, the kinds of problems which occurred in the research and agricultural animals such as bleeding, abnormal blood clots, failing hearts, low sperm counts and fertility issues and high cholesterol and atherosclerosis, are all problems that affect human beings. This review of studies presented above suggests that reducing cottonseed toxin intake will reduce risk of these kinds of problems.

CHAPTER 3

EXPANDING ON WHAT WE KNOW: COULD COTTONSEED CAUSE ALZHEIMER'S?

To this point, I have discussed what we already know about cottonseed toxins. We know that cottonseed toxins cause animals to die if fed in large enough doses. We know that the cottonseed toxin gossypol causes male sterility, and we know that cycloproprenoid fatty acids cause high cholesterol and atherosclerosis. The question that I asked was: if cottonseed toxins cause these problems in animals, could the toxins be causing the same and other problems in people? In this chapter, I describe how I came up with a hypothesis that might explain some of the causes of Alzheimer's. In the next chapter, I will describe my research that tests this hypothesis.

Using the current research as a starting point, I became interested in what might be a cause of Alzheimer's. Finding a cause of Alzheimer's is the first step toward preventing a terrible illness. Preventing a devastating illness is the best course of action. Because I am both a medical doctor (psychiatrist) and a Ph.D. nutritionist, I naturally tend to look at what people eat in relation to disease.

Why consider cottonseed toxins as a possible cause of Alzheimer's. Cottonseed toxins reach the brain.[21] Any toxic chemical which enters the brain could be considered as a possible cause of Alzheimer's. But there are other reasons to look at such toxins.

Cottonseed toxins cause similar problems to the medical findings in Alzheimer's

One first needs to understand something about the medical findings in Alzheimer's. Alzheimer's can be thought of as a problem in which people sadly lose their memory and have behavioral changes. However, Alzheimer's is not just a behavioral condition. The behavioral changes in Alzheimer's patients are associated with real physical changes in their brains. To be truly accurate, Alzheimer's can only be diagnosed by examining the patient's brain after death.

Alzheimer's findings in the brain

During life, however, doctors can observe changes in the brain in CT scans. The main observation is that the brain of Alzheimer's patients is smaller, containing less volume. Inside the brain are structures called ventricles that contain cerebrospinal fluid which protects the brain from damage due to physical trauma. In healthy young people, the ventricles appear very small on a CT scan. The brain takes up almost all the space, and the ventricles are small. In Alzheimer's patients, the ventricles appear very large because the brain, which surrounds the ventricles, has now shrunk. Why has the brain shrunk? Because brain cells have died and disappeared, leaving fewer cells which occupy less brain volume. Why might brain cells be dying in brain of Alzheimer's? Let us look more specifically at brain findings in Alzheimer's.

Pathologists, the doctors who study the brains in deceased Alzheimer's patients, find general deterioration of the brain and specific lesions or abnormalities in the brains of Alzheimer's patients. The main lesion which concerns us here is called the neurofibrillary tangle.

Neurofibrillary tangles are clumps of protein. A number of proteins make up neurofibrillary tangles and one of the main ones is called "tau." Neurofibrillary tangles are found in dead cells in the brain in Alzheimer's patients. Neurofibrillary tangles are actually clumps of several proteins including tau. In the normal brain, tau is part of the structure of microtubules, which makes up the skeleton of cells as explained in the last chapter. On microscope slides, in non-scientific terms, these neurofibrillary tangles look like messes of brown stuff. In scientific terms, they have a very characteristic appearance.

How might these neurofibrillary tangles form?

To explain further, most cells, including brain cells, have a structure called a "cytoskeleton" which forms the structure of the cell. Cytoskeletons are made of microtubules, which are made of proteins including tau and other proteins. Microtubules are like supporting beams in a large building; they hold up the structure, but are not visible under a microscope. Microtubules are called "in solution" when they are not visible. Each microtubule is far enough from the next microtubule that there is plenty of fluid between them. But in the brains of Alzheimer's patients, pathologists find clumps of insoluble microtubules. The microtubules do not have fluid separating them because they have collapsed together. These clumps of microtubules form "neurofibrillary tangles."

Cottonseed toxins and brain findings of Alzheimer's

Now let's go back to the existing research about cottonseed toxins. Brain cells and sperm cells both have microtubules. The cottonseed poison gossypol binds to microtubules in sperm and prevents the microtubules from organizing themselves normally. Gossypol prevents sperm from being formed, causing decreased sperm counts and ultimately male sterility in humans and animals.

If gossypol also were to bind to microtubules in brain cells, as it does in sperm cells, the gossypol could be deforming the microtubules.

Then the microtubules could become weak and collapse. When they collapse, they form neurofibrillary tangles such as one sees in Alzheimer's.

Gossypol binding to the cytoskeleton of the cell could also be causing cell death and decreased brain volume. Normal brain cytoskeletons do not spontaneously collapse. But if they are continually being weakened for years, they might collapse.

For these reasons alone, gossypol and cottonseed toxins should be tested as a possible cause of Alzheimer's disease.

Risk factors associated with Alzheimer's

In addition to current knowledge about changes in the brain in Alzheimer's, scientists also study Alzheimer's from a different perspective. Today, biomedical scientists do not what causes Alzheimer's. Without knowing the cause, scientists study conditions which may be associated with development of Alzheimer's. Scientists study these associated conditions hoping to learn something from the associated condition which may help scientists better understand the cause of the disease Alzheimer's. For example, scientists know from previous research studies that there are biological conditions known as risk factors associated with development of Alzheimer's. Scientists study these risk factors to see how they may contribute to the development of Alzheimer's. Ideally, scientists should also look at these risk factors to see whether toxic substances might contribute to the development of the biological conditions and risk factors which would in turn be associated with development of Alzheimer's.

The first risk factor is high cholesterol.[22] Scientists have identified high cholesterol as a risk factor by looking at who develops Alzheimer's and who does not. People with high cholesterol are more likely to develop Alzheimer's. This is an important association, not necessarily a cause. The exact reason for this association is not known at this time.

The second risk factor is what is called "microbleeding."[23] Researchers have observed in the brain in Alzheimer's patients, small areas of bleeding, which they term "microbleeding". These microbleeds are thought to be important in Alzheimer's. The bleeding may be important by itself or may trigger other events in the brain or both.

A third risk factor is a biological process thought to be important in Alzheimer's, increases in membrane permeability. Such changes allow chemicals to cross cell membranes, which ordinarily would not cross the membranes into the cell.[24] Such changes can prevent cells from doing their jobs properly. Again the mechanism for how these changes could lead to Alzheimer's is not known with certainty.

A fourth risk factor may be a lifestyle risk factor. Two studies have shown that increased meat intake is associated with an increased likelihood of developing Alzheimer's.[25]

Cottonseed causes all of the risk factors associated with Alzheimer's

Interestingly, cottonseed toxins cause all four of these risk factors. I have outlined in the previous chapter how cottonseed toxins cause increased cholesterol. Cottonseed toxins also cause bleeding, and changes in membrane permeability. These studies are well documented.

Finally, cottonseed toxins are stored in animal fats, including meat, and might explain why eating meat might raise the risk of developing Alzheimer's.

Cottonseed toxins cause all of the risk factors associated with Alzheimer's. Therefore, researching whether cottonseed toxins may be a cause of Alzheimer's is worthwhile, especially given high cottonseed toxicity and the pervasiveness of cottonseed toxins in the average diet.

Conclusion

I have shown in this chapter why I believe that scientists should research cottonseed toxins as a potential cause of Alzheimer's. This hypothesis is based on several observations. Cottonseed toxins are known to cause major health problems in animals. These problems include high cholesterol, atherosclerosis, bleeding disorders and heart failure. I explained in this chapter that all of these problems (except heart failure) are also known Alzheimer's risk factors. Therefore, researching whether cottonseed is a possible cause of Alzheimer's is valuable.

In addition to the risk factors, however, I have shown that scientists know that cottonseed toxins bind to microtubules in sperm.[26] In this chapter, I have shown how cottonseed toxin binding to microtubules in brain could lead to collapse of the cellular structure in brain. The brains of Alzheimer's patients, after death, show neurofibrillary tangles, which are made of collapsed microtubules. Another medical finding in Alzheimer's is smaller brain volume, which is a result of cells dying. One source of cells dying is from the collapse of the cellular structure, which is related to the same issues with microtubules. Therefore, since cottonseed toxins cause the same types of problems with microtubules in another area of the body, it is worth investigating whether cottonseed toxins cause the same problems with microtubules in the brain.

For collapse of the brain cellular structure to occur, cottonseed toxins must be present for a long period of time. This presence could only occur if cottonseed toxins accumulate instead of being cleared. This subject will be considered again in a later chapter.

Do cottonseed toxins accumulate? The third observation is that animals do not clear cottonseed toxins from their bodies.[27] If the animal could clear cottonseed toxins immediately, they would not be a problem. However animals do not clear all cottonseed toxins immediately. The cottonseed toxins remain in the animals. Then, when people eat meat from animals, they are consuming cottonseed toxins. In addition, if animals do not clear cottonseed toxins, one can reasonably assume that people also do not clear cottonseed toxin because people are similar to animals in how they metabolize toxins. Nothing in the literature suggests otherwise. Since animals fed cottonseed toxins gossypol and CPFA accumulate those toxins over their lifetimes, people would too. People eat cottonseed toxins over a much longer lifetime than those animals. People also consume cottonseed toxins both directly in cottonseed oil and indirectly in food such as meat and dairy. Nothing in the scientific literature suggests that people would accumulate CPFA or gossypol differently than animals.

Therefore, based on all of this information, I hypothesized that cottonseed toxins may be a cause of Alzheimer's.

To see how I tested this hypothesis, read on!

CHAPTER 4

MY EXPERIMENT FEEDING COTTONSEED TO RATS: HOW I FOUND THAT COTTONSEED CAUSES ALZHEIMER'S AND OTHER DISEASES

I have explained in the previous chapters that cottonseed is known to be toxic in large quantities in short term situations. The problem in real life, however, is that people eat much smaller quantities of the toxins over the course of many years. Scientists have not yet studied the effects of long term, lower level, exposure to cottonseed toxins, which is much more analogous to the human diet. I decided to test this long term, lower level exposure.

How I designed my experiment

What is the best design of an experiment to show the effects of long term ingestion of low levels of toxins? Seven significant issues had to be solved to design such an experiment.

First, one must remember that one cannot experiment on people without informed consent. Such experimentation is unethical and illegal if the point of the experiment is to feed toxic substances that could cause harmful effects. Therefore, one must determine what type of experiment would closely replicate the human experience. This experiment used an animal model. Female rats were used for reasons explained below.

Second, one must remember that eating lower levels of toxin over longer periods of time is exactly what human beings do. An experiment should replicate this human situation. Human beings live a long time during which time they ingest many toxins but most humans do not develop Alzheimer's until they have lived at least 70 or more years. So the feeding period has to be for a lifetime.

Third, in the human situation, toxins come in daily in small amounts. To replicate this situation, one would need to feed animals the toxins daily in small amounts over the lifetime of the animal.

Fourth, are the toxins separate from the diet or mixed into the diet? Poisons generally taste bad. Generally, human beings only eat things that taste bad because other more tasty parts of food mask the bad tasting items. Think about medicines such as antibiotics. Although medicine is not a poison, it tastes bad, and people won't take it unless flavorings mask the taste. For example pharmacists use a bubble gum flavor to mask the taste of amoxicillin for children. Similarly, animals do not eat pure poison if they have another choice. This is a survival technique! So an investigator needs either to mask the taste of the toxin, not offer a choice, or both. In the case of cottonseed, we found out in the early stages of this experiment that rats avoided eating any cottonseed when given the choice. This observation was interesting in itself but also meant that the cottonseed had to be mixed into the animals' food.

Answering these first four questions, we did the following. We mixed the cottonseed into the food at low levels. The animals only were offered this food. That way, they ate the toxins daily as part of their regular food intake.

We had three more questions to answer before actually starting the experiment.

Question five was, how should we determine what level of cottonseed to feed, based on the level of toxin in the actual human diet?

Again, we tried to replicate the human situation. How much cottonseed toxin do human beings eat? This question is considered in more detail in another chapter. For this experiment, we considered a study which showed the amount of the cottonseed toxin gossypol contained in a piece of chicken.[28] A piece of chicken contains four parts per million of the cottonseed poison gossypol. But human beings eat other things besides chicken. Some parts of the food supply contain more than four parts per million of gossypol, such as liver. Other foods, such as rice or vegetables, contain no cottonseed. Taking protein to be about 20% of the diet, and knowing that most predominantly protein containing foods, such as meat or fish, contain cottonseed poison, we determined that an average intake of cottonseed poison might be 20% of 4 ppm or about 0.8 ppm. Based on this information, we used 1 ppm gossypol, rounding up from 0.8 ppm.

Question six was, which animal would be most appropriate for this experiment? The answer to this question depended in part on the sensitivity of different animals to toxins. In earlier studies, rabbits were quite sensitive to cottonseed toxins and rats were less sensitive. No one knows exactly how sensitive human beings are to cottonseed. If human beings and rats are equally sensitive to cottonseed toxin, then feeding the approximate human intake of cottonseed toxin to rats would be most appropriate. What though, if the animals, in this case, female rats, were more or less sensitive to cottonseed poison than humans? If one chooses a level of toxin to feed, and the level is too low to show an effect, then the experiment is worthless. If one chooses a level of toxin to feed, and the level is too high, the experiment can be criticized for not replicating the human situation. We resolved this problem by feeding primarily the same level as estimated for human beings, but adding an experimental group which received ten times the amount of toxins. If rats are less sensitive to cottonseed toxin than humans, a level of intake ten times higher than that of humans should still be enough to bring out an effect if such an effect is present.

In this experiment, 1 ppm of gossypol (an estimation of human intake) was fed in several different forms but an additional group of animals was fed 10 ppm of gossypol in the form of whole cottonseed. Rats were chosen because their lifetime at two and a half to three years is short enough for a lifetime study. Rats are also commonly used to study human problems because the physiology of rats is similar to that of human beings. Rats on average live two years, up to almost three years. We further chose female rats because they live on average longer than male rats. Using female rats, on average, maximized the exposure to cottonseed over a course of a lifetime.

The seventh, and final question, is which form of cottonseed to use?

Researching cottonseed is complicated because there is not only one cottonseed toxin. As I explained in previous chapters, cottonseed contains many different toxins. The toxins are also not all in the same place in the cottonseed. None are in the hull. Some toxins end up in the oil, and some end up in meal, which is the part remaining after pressing out the oil. So cottonseed in several different forms must be fed to see the effects of all the toxins acting together and at least partially separately.

Whole cottonseed contains all the poisons, including gossypol, the cyclopropenoid fatty acids and the poisons which have not been well studied. The oil contains the cyclopropenoid fatty acids, which are associated with high cholesterol and heart and artery disease problems. Other poisons including gossypol will be in the cottonseed meal. Gossypol is only one of these poisons. We don't know much about the rest.

If we feed only gossypol to rats, we could miss the effects of the other poisons which have not yet been researched. The only way to find out the effects of the other poisons is to feed the cottonseed meal to some animals and to feed whole cottonseed to some animals.

Cottonseed comes commercially in several forms. Cottonseed is found as cottonseed meal, which contains minimal oil, because most of it has been pressed out. Cottonseed comes also comes as whole cottonseed. Cottonseed oil is also used industrially. For this experiment, I had to purchase cottonseed. Cottonseed is not on a typical list of scientific research products. So I had to purchase the cottonseed that was available commercially, mostly to farmers. To purchase the cottonseed, I went to a feed store to buy it. I had much more difficulty with obtaining cottonseed oil. I was unable to purchase cottonseed oil because it is only sold in large industrial quantities. I could not use cottonseed oil that is available in the stores for average consumers because the purity of the oil was unreliable. I was able to purchase cottonseed meal from an agricultural supplier. Small amounts of gossypol are available from a scientific supplier.

Experimental Design: Groups of Animals

Now that we answered the major questions, we were able to design an experiment to test my hypothesis that cottonseed toxins might be a cause of Alzheimer's in people.

In this experiment, we used 65 rats, divided into five groups of 13 each. These groups were as follows:

- ✓ **Group 1: "Control Group"** This group of animals received a regular diet with no cottonseed. Recall that in any good scientific study, one must have a control group that receives only the regular diet. Otherwise, one does not know whether any results are due to the regular diet or whether the toxins have any effect.

- ✓ **Group 2: "CSM Group"** This group received the regular diet plus cottonseed meal at 0.058% of the diet. ("CSM group" stands for cottonseed meal group). This amount of cottonseed meal has gossypol sufficient for 1 ppm in the entire CSM diet.

✓ **Group 3: "WCS 1"** This group received the regular diet plus whole cottonseed at 0.013% of the diet (WCS stands for "whole cottonseed"; since this is the first WCS group, it is called WCS 1). This amount of whole cottonseed has gossypol sufficient for 1 ppm in the entire WCS 1 diet.

✓ **Group 4: "GOSS"** This group received the regular diet plus pure gossypol (the "GOSS" group, standing for gossypol). The pure gossypol was 1 ppm of the entire GOSS diet.

✓ **Group 5: "WCS 2"** This group received the regular diet plus 10 times as much as whole cottonseed as WCS 1, or 0.13% of the diet. The amount of gossypol they received was 10 ppm, instead of 1 ppm.

✓ As stated above, the "CSM group," the "whole cottonseed 1" group (WCS 1) and the "GOSS group" were all receiving the toxin gossypol in the amount of about 1 ppm of the diet. But the gossypol group only received gossypol, with no other toxins mixed in. The "CSM group" received all the cottonseed poisons found in cottonseed meal, including gossypol. The group "whole cottonseed 1" group received all the cottonseed poisons including gossypol and the cyclopropenoid fatty acids.

✓ The reason for including the WCS 2 group, receiving 10 times the amount of cottonseed, was to make sure that if there were effects of cottonseed poisons that were only found at higher amounts, those effects would be seen. 10 ppm exposure is two and a half times the amount found in a piece of chicken. Even at ten ppm, the amount of whole cottonseed fed to rats is much less than the amounts used in prior agricultural experiments.

What did we expect?

As all good scientists do, we started with a hypothesis. The hypothesis was that dietary cottonseed toxins cause problems such as bleeding, Alzheimer's and heart disease. Even though a review of prior studies suggested this hypothesis may be correct, there was still a possibility such problems would not be seen in our experiment. In some of the few toxicology studies done on cottonseed, rats were found to be less sensitive to cottonseed poisons than other species such as rabbits.

We did not know whether we would observe results in rats, because most of the studies in cottonseed toxin studies, such as heart disease and bleeding, were done on other kinds of animals. Rats do not normally develop any form of heart disease as they age. In addition, rats have never been shown to develop any Alzheimer's lesions. In general, human neurological disorders are seldom seen in animals. Rats, however, have been shown to bleed when gossypol is given by injection. From this perspective, we might have expected to find little if we fed small amounts of cottonseed to rats for a lifetime. Any findings of heart disease or Alzheimer's would be very significant.

Thus, we started the experiment knowing that we had little chance of results. We also would not know what our results were until after the animals had all died naturally. Alzheimer's is diagnosed by pathology on the brain after death. We did not do any memory studies on the rats as we went along. Therefore, we had no basis to suspect which rats might or might not have brain lesions that indicated Alzheimer's. Instead, we fed the rats over the course of their natural lifetime, preserved them after death and waited until all of the animals had died. Then we found out what illnesses or diseases they had.

What did we find?

The experimental results were very important. We found that by feeding rats small amounts of cottonseed, we produced many of the diseases affecting mankind in the western world. Feeding cottonseed and cottonseed poison at seemingly low levels over a lifetime was not benign. Major physical abnormalities and signs of disease (pathologies) were found as the rats aged. A level of poison which was easily tolerated for a few months in young rats had devastating effects as those rats became older.

Bleeding Disorders, Aneurysms and Atherosclerosis

We found no evidence of atherosclerosis or Alzheimer's in the control group (the rats that did not receive any cottonseed).

But other problems developed in rats fed cottonseed. In the rats fed cottonseed meal (CSM), we observed based on one animal's behavior while alive that the animal appeared to have had a stroke. This rat seemed off balance and could not move one side of its body. We did not change the experiment; we only noted this behavior. After this rat died, we were able to examine its brain. We found that this rat had suffered two intracerebral hemorrhages (areas of bleeding in the brain). These were in two separate areas of the brain. This finding alone is important because there has never been a report of an intracerebral hemorrhage (bleeding stroke) in a normal aging rat.

In the group of rats fed whole cottonseed at 0.013% of the diet (WCS-I), one animal developed atherosclerosis in the aorta. Atherosclerosis may be found in any artery, from the coronary arteries feeding the heart to the large aorta. Both are found in humans. The reason investigators look for atherosclerosis in the rat aorta is that the rat aorta is big enough to see such atherosclerosis easily. Another rat in this group, a WCS-I rat, suffered a major kidney hemorrhage. Again, these findings are significant because the scientific literature contains no reports of major kidney hemorrhages in aging rats. There are also no reports of atherosclerosis in aging rats in the scientific literature. The WCS-I group of animals received whole cottonseed, which contains all the cottonseed poisons including the cyclopropenoid fatty acids and gossypol. Again, none of the rats in the control group had these diseases.

In the group of rats fed whole cottonseed (WCS-II), at 0.13% of the diet (ten times that of WCS-1), we found several major health problems. Three of the rats (out of 13), which is 23% of the total group, had atherosclerosis (coronary artery disease but in the aorta). The atherosclerotic plaques in two of the rats were of moderate severity and the third was very severe, likely enough to have caused death. In the third rat, the more severe abnormality contained a large atherosclerotic plaque which had ulcerated. This means that the plaque had literally broken open, and was bleeding into an aortic aneurysm, which is a major weakening of the wall of the aorta. Aortic aneurysm is a common problem in human beings but the cause of such aneurysms in humans has not been understood previously.

Like the findings of major kidney hemorrhages, atherosclerosis, and intra-cerebral hemorrhages, the scientific literature contains no reports of aortic aneurysm in any animal, including rats.

So at this point, we have not one, not two, not three, but four major health problems that occurred only in the rats fed cottonseed toxins: kidney hemorrhages, atherosclerosis, intra-cerebral hemorrhages and aortic aneurysm.

To review: there were 39 female rats which ate either cottonseed meal or whole cottonseed, and an additional 13 rats that ate a diet containing 1 ppm gossypol. We had 13 rats in a control group that did not receive cottonseed in either form or gossypol. Out of the 39 rats which ate some form of cottonseed, we found four with major bleeds, one in the kidney, two in the brain and one in the aorta. Out of 13 rats which ate higher levels of whole cottonseed, we found that three rats had atherosclerosis. One of 13 rats which ate the lower level of whole cottonseed had aortic atherosclerosis. To repeat, these are completely new findings. None of these disorders have been reported in aging animals of any species. None of these disorders were found in the control group.

One way scientists evaluate how significant experimental findings are is by asking if the findings could have occurred by chance. Findings which could have occurred by chance are much less significant than findings which are extremely unlikely to have occurred by chance. There is no way in a study with only a modest number of animals that four bleeding events such as we found could occur by chance. These events occurred because these animals were fed cottonseed. Moreover, this finding is similar to studies of animals (presented in prior chapters) which have been fed larger amounts of cottonseed. Scientists have demonstrated that larger short term amounts of cottonseed cause bleeding. What our experiment showed is that small amounts of cottonseed over long periods of time cause bleeding.

The study also showed that the small amounts of cottonseed fed over long periods of time caused atherosclerosis. These findings have never been reported in normally aging rats. Such findings are consistent with studies presented earlier that dietary cottonseed toxins cause atherosclerosis in rabbits. These atherosclerotic plaques in rats are due to feeding cottonseed toxins.

Alzheimer's findings

Did any of the rats show findings of Alzheimer's?

In all of the groups of animals which received cottonseed or gossypol in the diet, including the final group which received pure gossypol at 1 ppm (GOSS), we found Alzheimer's lesions. We did not find any Alzheimer's lesions in the control group which received no cottonseed or gossypol.

We noted earlier that the basic lesion of Alzheimer's under a microscope slide of the brain is dark brown staining material inside cells termed "neurofibrillary tangles." Such lesions are seen, although they can be hard to find, in the brains of older people who had Alzheimer's. Such lesions, however, have only been reported a handful of times in a few animals, and never in rats. These lesions were described in humans more than one hundred years ago and continue to be seen today under a light microscope.

We found what appeared to be neurofibrillary tangles, the same dark brown staining material that has been observed for 100 years in Alzheimer's patients after death. We found the highest concentration of these lesions in the group of rats fed the higher level of whole cottonseed (WCS 2). But every group that was fed some cottonseed or gossypol showed some animals with some such lesions. These differences will be explained in a later chapter.

We primarily looked for Alzheimer's lesions in the oldest rats, the rats which lived a full life span (some rats had died earlier due to other causes of death, which are common in laboratory rats). We examined only the oldest rats due to expense, and also due to the greater likelihood of finding Alzheimer's lesions in older rats due to the nature of the illness, which is a disease associated with aging.

The results are as follows:

We took the six oldest rats in the control group (days of survival, 771 to 948 days). We did not find any neurofibrillary tangles. In the other groups, we also looked at the oldest rats. In CSM, there were four rats examined with the same age parameters. Two of the four, showed neurofibrillary tangles (1027 and 1081 days of survival). In WCS-I, which was the group of lower-level cottonseed, one of three older rats showed neurofibrillary tangles (days of survival 930). In WCS-II, the higher level of whole cottonseed, all of the older animals had neurofibrillary tangles. That is, the five rats who lived the longest, (868 to 1030 days survival), had a 100% rate of neurofibrillary tangles. In the GOSS group, which were rats fed 1 ppm pure gossypol, the oldest four rats (889 to 1081 days survival), had a rate of 75% showing neurofibrillary tangles. That is, three of the four oldest gossypol fed rat brains showed neurofibrillary tangles. In general, larger numbers of neurofibrillary tangles were observed in the rats fed whole cottonseed at the higher level and the next larger numbers were observed in the gossypol (GOSS) fed rats.

These rats developed neurofibrillary tangles, a classic sign of Alzheimer's disease, from being fed small amounts of cottonseed every day for their lifetimes.

If you would like to see the actual pictures of what this looks like, please look at the end of this chapter and go to our website, at http://wisresearch.com.

Another significant point is that just like the other four major findings that I discussed above, the scientific literature contains no reports of a normally aging rat developing neurofibrillary tangles. The only reports are in rats that have genetically manipulated to contain faulty genes to allow scientists to study Alzheimer's. I did not use such rats. I used normal laboratory rats.

These findings were astonishing. Even in a very small group of animals, we created a high rate of life altering disease by feeding low levels of cottonseed toxins over a lifetime, designed to reproduce the human situation. This was not a study like previous cottonseed studies, which created major problems in animals by feeding higher levels of cottonseed toxins short term. We expected that the scientific community would be interested in these findings. Potentially, people could control for themselves a very large risk factor for life altering diseases, including Alzheimer's, heart disease and stroke.

Initially, I submitted the above findings for publication but was met with simple disbelief on the part of the scientific reviewers. I explain the process of publication in a later chapter, and how that process affects the ability to do scientific research and to get that information to the public. Part of the issue, it appeared, was that the reviewers wanted more precise indicators of Alzheimer's before they would consider the possibility that dietary cottonseed toxin was actually related to disease in the brain. The microscopic finding of a neurofibrillary tangle is not considered a precise enough indicator in current Alzheimer's research. Such a more precise indicator of the steps in the Alzheimer's disease process is called "phosphorylated tau". The presence of phosphorylated tau is considered to be a major step in the Alzheimer's disease process. I decided to pursue further research to determine if we could detect "phosphorylated tau," a major marker of Alzheimer's only evident with special preparation (again, after death). Unfortunately, special chemistry, available to a few researchers in University labs, is required to determine the presence of phosphorylated tau. My lab was not equipped for this type of work. After efforts were made to find a researcher who could perform such studies, a researcher at a major university expressed interest in this experiment. We sent her some of the microscopic sections (slides) for evaluation for phosphorylated tau. She and her lab did indeed find phosphorylated tau. So even by today's more exacting standards, we had in fact found Alzheimer's Disease in these animals. However, this researcher was not interested in pursuing the research further, or in publication of these findings, so those findings have not been published with complete details.

Other Brain Findings

In addition to Alzheimer's, we found other brain abnormalities. Most of the old rats had developed a problem in their brains called "mucoid globules." These are named because they look like clusters of grapes under the microscope. In reality, mucoid globules are dying brain cells. They were first described in 1923, and have been found in Alzheimer's and Parkinson's Disease. Mucoid globules actually have never been reported in normal aging animals.

Unlike some other problems that we are discussing, we also found mucoid globules in some of the control rats which did not receive any cottonseed. In the control rats, we found the mucoid globules in only one limited area of the brain. It is possible that mucoid globules are part of aging. However, the location of the mucoid globules is very significant. Unlike the control rats, the rats which received the most cottonseed developed mucoid globules throughout deep areas of the brain, not just in one limited area of the brain. The control rats did not show lesions deep in the more important structures of the brain. These mucoid globules indicate a problem with dying cells throughout the brain in the cottonseed fed rats, not just in one limited area of the brain.

In addition to mucoid globules, we saw evidence in the oldest rats which were fed cottonseed, that the mucoid globules themselves were older. In other words, brain cell death may have been occurring earlier in the cottonseed fed rats. When brain cells die, first there is a mucoid globule. Then the mucoid globule dissolves and disappears, leaving a hole. We found large holes in the brain, which resulted from the mucoid globules dissolving and disappearing. So not only were mucoid globules present in deeper areas of the brains of the rats which ate cottonseed, but they appeared to have developed sooner, and collapsed, leaving large holes where brain tissue had once been. Abnormalities such as mucoid globules and large holes in the brain indicate that cottonseed causes a general deterioration of the brain, not just neurofibrillary tangles. Mucoid globules are also associated with development of Parkinson's disease.

Atherosclerosis, aneurysms, Alzheimer's and more general brain deterioration as indicated by holes in the brain are all problems which develop over long periods of time. This is consistent with a low level poison acting slowly over a lifetime.

What is the Meaning for Us?

My experiment has major implications for all of us, which I will explain in greater detail in the next chapter. My experiment showed that small amounts of cottonseed caused Alzheimer's, atherosclerosis, bleeding problems, intracerebral hemorrhage (a type of stroke), and aortic aneurysm. The animals in my experiment ate an amount of cottonseed comparable to the average human diet. This is the first reported study ever showing all of these effects in animals fed at low levels over the course of their lifetime.

What does this mean for us? Keep reading.

On the next pages are pictures of some of the findings. Some of the pictures are from normal animals for comparison. Figure 1 is from a normal rat brain. In normal brain, there are areas of cells and other areas of nerve cell fibers, which makes for different looking areas. Figure 2 is from a rat fed cottonseed meal in which many cells have died, leaving many holes in the brain. Figure 3 is another photograph of normal rat brain. Figure 4 is a picture of an intracerebral hemorrhage, or in other words, a bleed into the brain. In human beings this would also be called a bleeding stroke. Figure 5 is a photograph of a normal brain using a silver stain. This is a stain special for nerve cells. Figure 6 is a picture of a collection of neurofibrillary tangles, from a rat fed the higher level of cottonseed. Figures 7 and 8 are closer views of neurofibrillary tangles from the same animal as shown in figure 6. Figure 9 is a single neurofibrillary tangle from a rat fed gossypol.

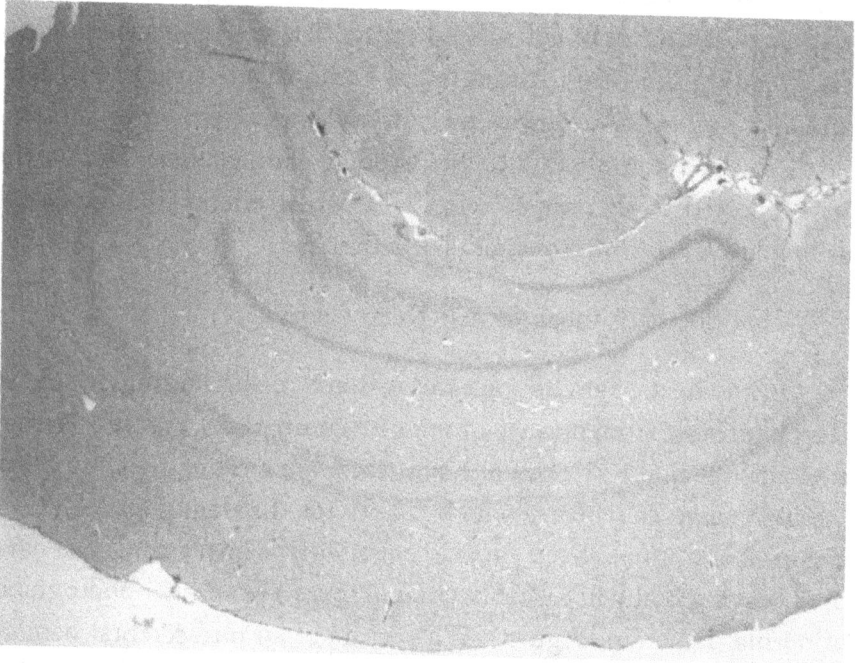

Figure 1: Normal rat brain

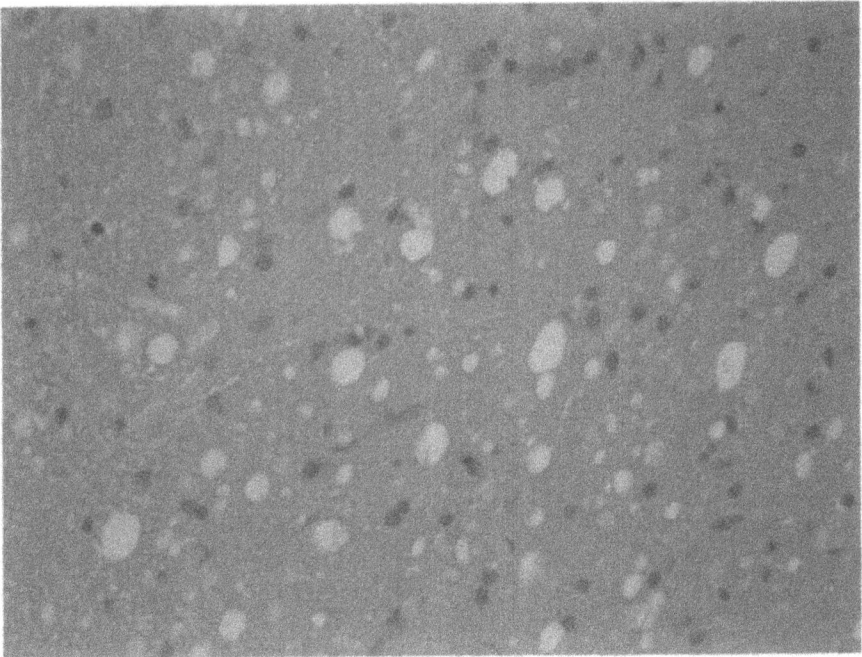

Figure 2: Brain from a rat fed cottonseed meal in which many cells have died, leaving many holes in the brain

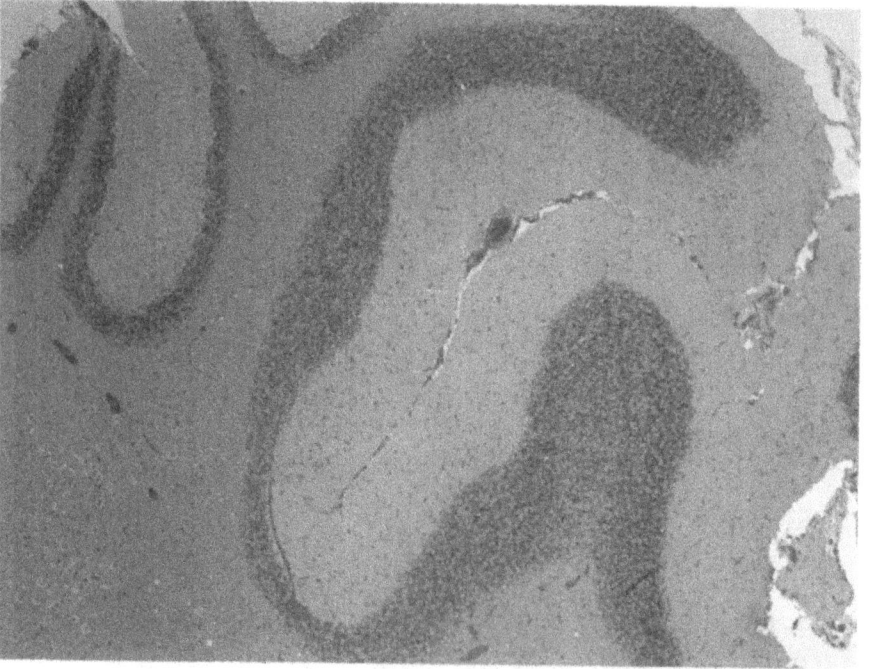

Figure 3: Normal rat brain

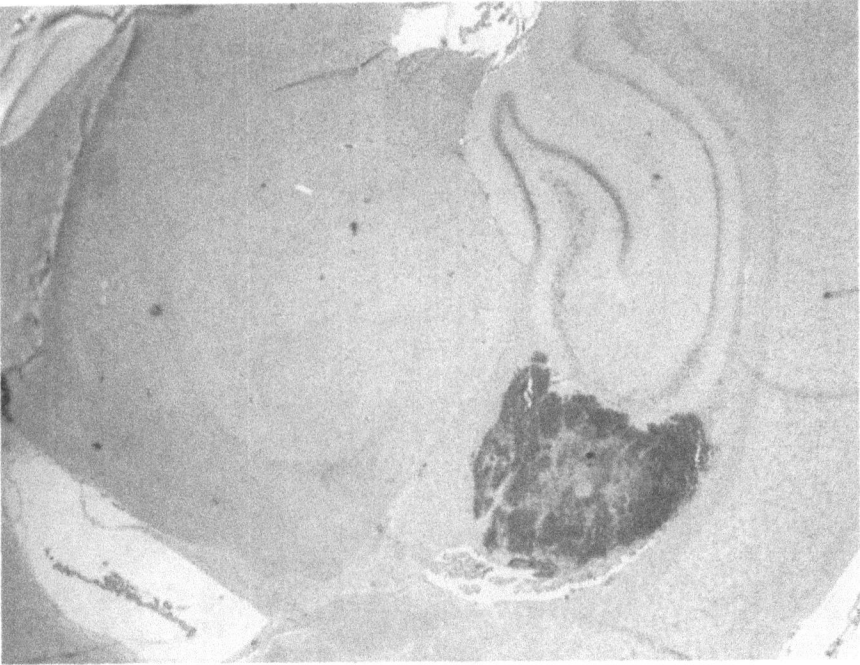

Figure 4: Picture of an intracerebral hemorrhage, or in other words,
a bleed into the brain

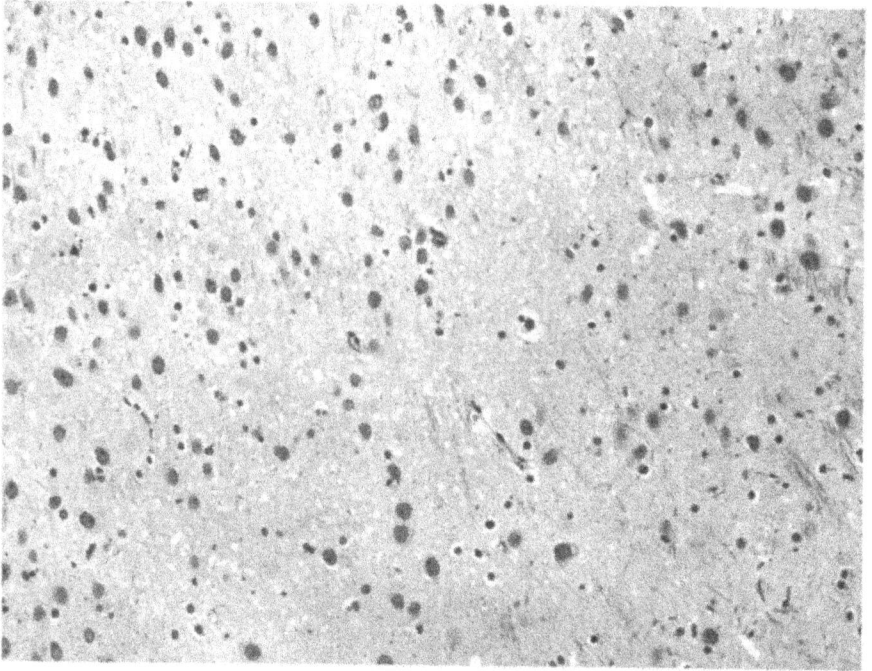

Figure 5: Photograph of a normal brain using a silver stain
(used to show neurofibrillary tangles)

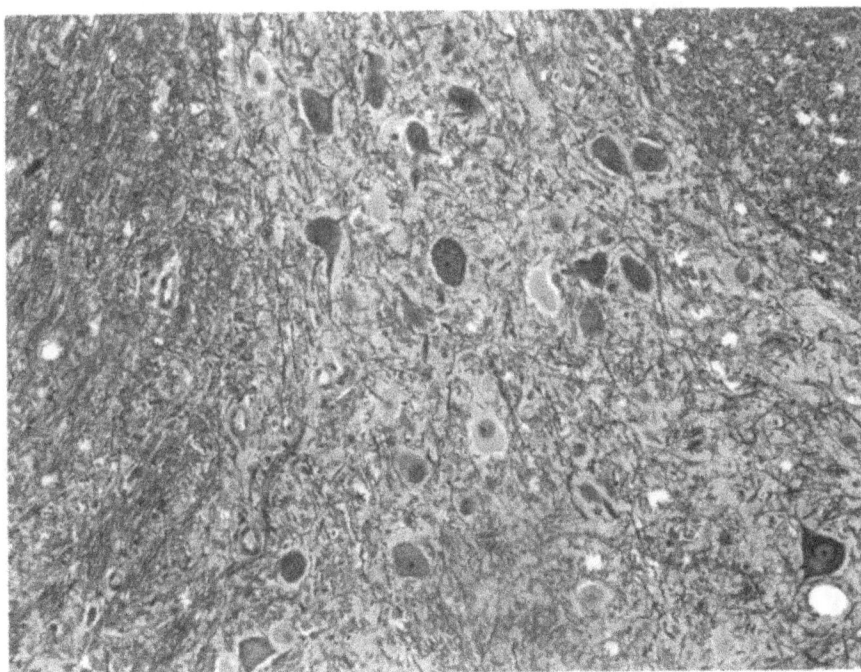

Figure 6: Picture in brain of a collection of neurofibrillary tangles, from a rat fed the higher level of cottonseed

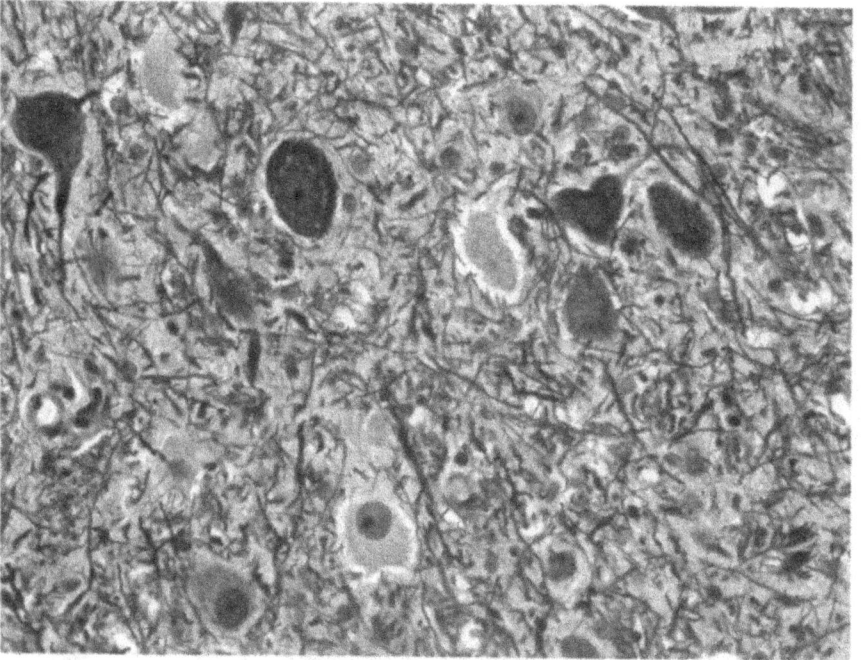

Figure 7: Closer view of neurofibrillary tangles from the same
animal as shown in figure 6

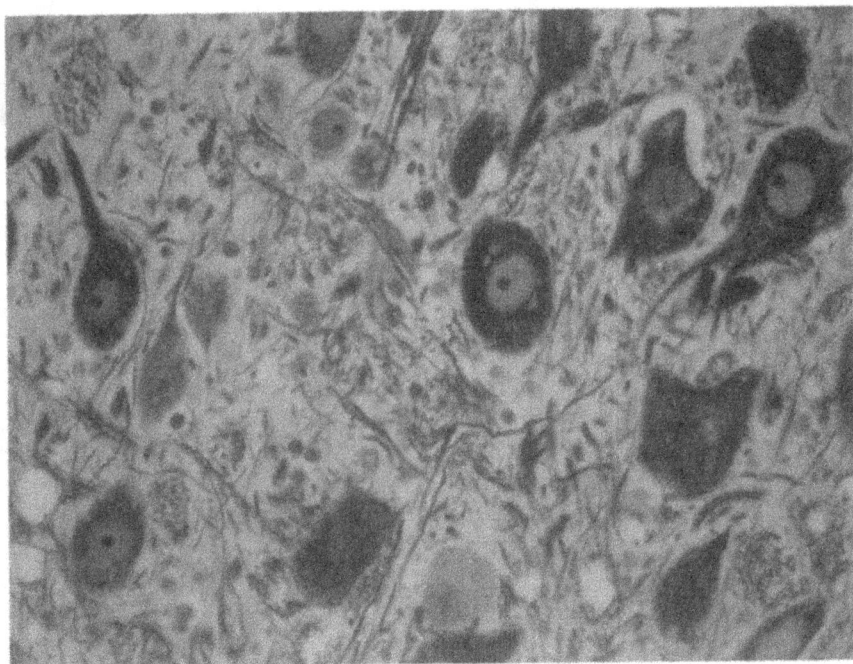

Figure 8: Closer view of neurofibrillary tangles from the
same animal as shown in figure 6

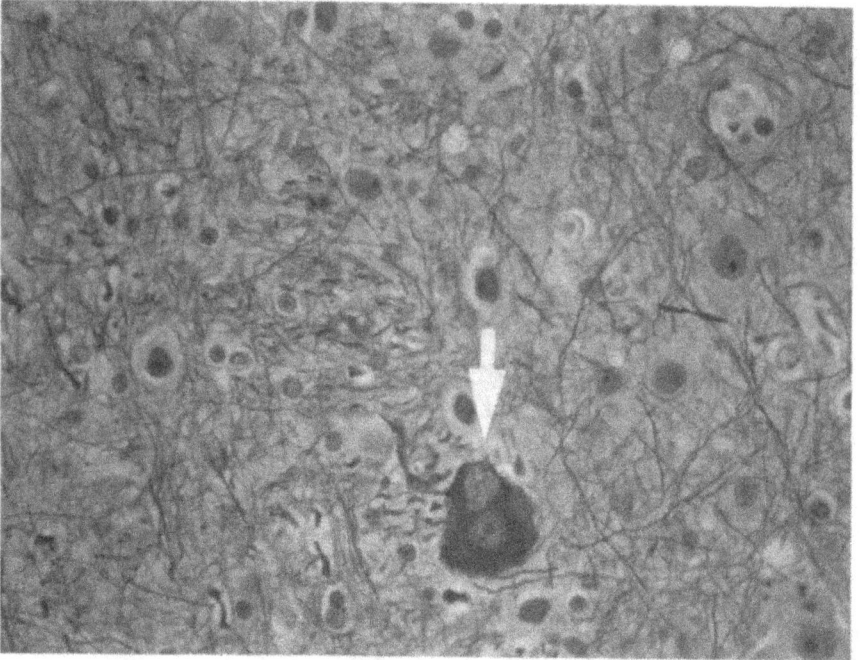

Figure 9: A single neurofibrillary tangle from brain of a rat fed gossypol.

CHAPTER 5

SHOULD YOU WORRY ABOUT EATING COTTONSEED? YES!

I just explained that when I fed rats various forms of cottonseed, they developed bleeding in their brains and other places, heart disease, and signs of Alzheimer's in brain.

So what? What does this study mean for you? Should you care?

Yes.

If I were in your situation—and I am—reading this information, I would ask myself whether eating food containing cottonseed toxins was worth the risk of developing Alzheimer's and these other major life threatening health problems.

For me and for my family, the convenience of eating foods containing cottonseed toxins is not worth the long-term risk of developing these problems. To reduce the risk of developing Alzheimer's and heart disease, I would advise, as a doctor, a nutritionist and a consumer, that everyone should avoid cottonseed, both in the direct form as oil and indirectly through meat, fish, poultry and dairy that is fed cottonseed. The reason is that the amounts of cottonseed that I used to feed the rats, which caused major health problems, are comparable to the amount of cottonseed toxins that people eat in everyday life. Let me explain.

Amount of cottonseed in the average human diet

People may argue that cottonseed is safe because people eat so "little" of it. After all, people do not consume cottonseed as a main or side dish. Think about it. Cottonseed is not even a food. It is an additive that became part of our food production because it is a waste product from cotton production, and cotton farmers saw a way to make a profit from this waste. Cottonseed oil appears as an ingredient in other foods, and cottonseed is a hidden ingredient in meat, fish and poultry.

If you are skeptical, I can understand why. People hear about studies showing that some food or food ingredient is bad for them in large quantities, and they think to themselves, if scientists use huge amounts of toxin to test for harmful effects, then the toxins must only be bad for people in huge amounts.

This is not that type of study. This is a realistic study. I did not use huge amounts of toxins. I used approximately the same amount of cottonseed toxins as people eat in everyday life. I took tremendous care to replicate the human situation. I did this because I wanted the study to be a real example of everyday life. I was not looking for dramatic results, but found them anyway. That is why this study is so critical. Eating quantities of cottonseed comparable to what normal people eat over their lifetimes, the rats developed evidence of Alzheimer's and other major brain and body diseases that are life-threatening in people.

So are the amounts of cottonseed in the human diet really comparable to the amounts used in this study? In the case of cyclopropenoid fatty acids, no one has ever measured the amount of cyclopropenoid fatty acids in human food as a whole, as a total. In the case of gossypol, there are measurements of the amounts in meat and other organs of farm animals but there are actually no official measurements of gossypol in food. One of the hardest steps in understanding the effects of dietary toxins is going from a toxicity study to real recommendations for people.

The question here is how much of a risk people are taking by eating foods containing cottonseed toxins. In the next few pages, I will do my best to explain the cottonseed toxin amounts present in human food. Because no one has made official measurements, my attempts may seem confusing. Yet for the sake of completeness, these explanations are necessary.

I am going to explain how I derived this information on toxin amounts in the diet. I calculated these dietary number for both gossypol and cyclopropenoid fatty acids (CPFA's). I explain the calculation of gossypol below.

This requires a lot of numbers, so bear with me please. If you want to skip the math, that's OK. Skip the next two sections, labeled "Math 1" and "Math 2" then come back to this chapter. The bottom line is that I calculated conservatively for gossypol and very conservatively for CPFA's. My goal was to not feed the rats more toxins than humans eat. My goal was to see if feeding the animals about the same amount as in the human diet would have an impact on their health. This is really the only way to help people assess whether they want to take the risk of continuing to eat cottonseed.

I used an approximation of gossypol that is actually present in the human diet, which works out to be about 1 part per million, which is about a half milligram per day of gossypol. I used the conservative amount of CPFA's, at approximately an eighth of the amount that an average person might consume. Even with numbers that do not exceed the content of the human diet, I found startling results, with enormous implications for our health.

Math 1: How I figured out how much Gossypol is in the average human diet

Here is the math for gossypol content in the human diet.

By the early 1960's, scientists developed measurement techniques to determine how much gossypol was present in the muscle and other tissues of animals fed cottonseed.[29] The first such report was done with pigs. The amount of gossypol found in muscle was about 4 to 8 ppm (parts per million). The muscle has some of the smallest amounts of all of the organs tested. The liver contained 10 times the amount found in muscle. Kidneys also had large amounts but less than in liver. This study also showed that gossypol was reaching the brain which had a little more than muscle at about 8 ppm.[30]

In a piece of chicken breast, the cottonseed toxin gossypol is present at about 4 parts per million (ppm). This number comes from the study done by Gamboa (2001). Gamboa (2001) fed cottonseed meal to broiler chickens at varying levels, up to 28% of the diet, for a total of 42 days.[31] Gamboa looked at how much gossypol was found in the tissues after death. In the breast muscle, they found between 2 and 5 ppm. In heart muscle, they found about four times that amount, or 16 ppm. In liver, they found at least ten times the amount found in breast muscle, or 40 ppm.

To put that number of 4 ppm in perspective, federal regulations allow the extremely toxic pesticide malathion to be present at only 8 ppm in fruit. Malathion is something people clear out of their bodies. Malathion is excreted within hours.[32] Malathion does not accumulate.

Nobody has ever done a study to show that the toxin gossypol is safe for people at 4 ppm. Remember, too, that 4 ppm is much lower than the amount found in the heart and livers of chicken.

The next factor to remember is that people do not only eat chicken. Other foods may have differing amounts of cottonseed toxin. So one can't be sure that 4 ppm is the actual amount of cottonseed people are consuming. One needs to look at other sources of cottonseed toxins. Recall that in a previous chapter I discussed that farmers feed cottonseed to chickens, pigs, farm fed fish and cattle. Studies show that all of these animals have 4 ppm or higher of gossypol in their muscle, which is the part of the animal that we commonly eat.

Based on the Gamboa study, an average person eats about 4 ppm of gossypol in the protein part of their diet. We know that most people eat protein at about 20% of the diet. This would mean that people might be taking in about 0.8 ppm of gossypol in all of their food. For the purpose of my study of feeding rats gossypol and cottonseed, I rounded up 0.8 ppm to 1 ppm. The estimate may be conservative, because some foods contain much more cottonseed toxins than other foods. For example, beef liver contains 20 times the amount of cottonseed toxins, about 80 ppm, and beef heart contains 10 times the amount of cottonseed toxins, about 40 ppm.[33] The estimated amount of gossypol in the diet may be higher than 0.8 or 1 ppm.

So, that explains how I derived the 1 ppm number. But it is not the end of the issue. Next one needs to consider that food safety is not a static, or one time, event. If people only ate cottonseed once, and the body cleared—or got rid of—the toxins, cottonseed might not be a problem. People might not need to worry at all about 1 ppm in all of our food.

However, the problem is that there is no reason to believe that people are able to clear cottonseed toxins any better than animals. Cottonseed toxins are hard to clear.

Poisons which accumulate are far worse than poisons (such as malathion) which are cleared immediately. For example, the human body clears ethyl alcohol. However, all of the animal studies show that animals do not clear cottonseed toxins. The toxins accumulate in their muscles and in their fat. The reason so much cottonseed toxin is found in liver is that the liver is a main organ for excreting toxins. Because the liver cannot easily clear the cottonseed toxin gossypol, much is found there.

Scientists studied gossypol separately from cyclopropenoid fatty acids (one of the other main cottonseed toxins). Both sets of studies show the same thing: cottonseed toxins accumulate. When researchers fed cottonseed meal to fish, the amount of gossypol found in the fish tissue continues to go up.[34] The fish cannot clear all the gossypol even if the researchers stop the cottonseed feeding. When a large amount of gossypol (traceable through radioactive markers) is given in one quick dose to an animal, some but not all of the gossypol is excreted.[35] Gossypol is found in all the major tissues and organs including the brain in pigs which are fed cottonseed meal.[36] We know from other studies that other toxins, including cyclopropenoid fatty acids, accumulate in the fat of every animal in which they have been tested, including rats and rabbits and in fish.[37]

Cottonseed is not only fed to chickens, pigs and fish. Farmers feed large amounts of cottonseed to beef and dairy cattle. Dairy cattle can be fed up to 10 percent whole cottonseed. The amount of gossypol present in the blood of a lactating dairy cow is very high, about 3000 ppm. Scientists don't know how much crosses the placenta and ends up in the milk, but even just 1% would be much more than the amount found in chicken.

I explained earlier that pigs, cows, chickens, and farmed fish which eat commercial feed all eat cottonseed toxins as a regular part of their diet. I explained earlier that scientists calculated the amount of cottonseed they could feed the animals before the cottonseed killed them. Based on these studies, a pig can be fed 100 ppm per day of gossypol as part of its feed over its lifetime. In contrast, human beings eat about 1% of the 100 ppm or about 1 ppm of gossypol in our regular diets.

The question is, how long would it take a human being to eat the same amount as the pig does over the course of a lifetime?

A pig is fed for about nine months to reach market size. Nine months is the average lifespan of the commercial pig. The average lifespan of a human being is much longer than the lifespan of a commercial pig. However, calculating the total amounts of gossypol consumed over the lifetime of a pig and the lifetime of a human surprisingly comes out to be about the same. Human beings take in the cottonseed toxins over a much longer period of time but the total amount of intake is approximately the same. Remember that humans eat about 1 ppm of cottonseed toxins daily, which is 1% of what the pigs consume daily but human beings consume the toxins for perhaps 100 times as long, for the same total accumulation and intake. The course of a human lifetime of consumption of cottonseed toxin may be 100 times the lifespan of a pig, or 100 times nine months, which comes out to be 900 months. 900 months is 75 years.

Think about what happens at about 75 years of age. This is a time when many people have developed health problems such as heart disease, and stroke. Many people unfortunately develop Alzheimer's around this age. I pose this question, is this a coincidence?

Math 2: How I figured out how much CPFA's are in the Human Diet

Cottonseed is complex because it contains a number of poisons which can lead to different diseases. I explained how gossypol causes problems. I also discussed how cyclopropenoid fatty acids (CPFA's) cause disease. This section is for the readers who want to know the quantity of CPFA's used in the experiment, which led to atherosclerosis. Understanding these numbers helps a reader understand the relative risk in the human diet. The question is are there enough CPFA in the human diet to cause coronary artery disease.

CPFA's become part of the human diet both directly and indirectly. The main source of CPFA's is cottonseed oil, which is used in cooking and food preparation. Other sources include indirect consumption through meat and dairy.

More specifically, what are the sources of CPFA's in the human diet? The first is cottonseed oil. Whole cottonseed is 16% cottonseed oil.ii Cottonseed oil contains 1 to 2% CPFA's.[38] So how much CPFA are in some common foods. There are no published amounts so we have to make calculations, which require some mathematics.

Let us look at doughnuts as an example of how to figure out the amount of CPFA's in the diet. Most doughnuts are fried. Doughnuts vary in size. For example, let us make this calculation for a commercially available doughnut. Keep in mind that this is just an example. A French Cruller at Dunkin Donuts, a national doughnut chain, is a 40 gram doughnut. It contains 250 calories. 20 grams of those calories are fat (180 calories), which is 30% of the donut. Some unknown percentage of this fat is cottonseed oil. Other oils include palm oil and soy oil.[39] This is just an example showing you how much cottonseed oil may be in the average diet.

Cottonseed oil makes up about 5 % of the vegetable oil in United States.[40]

According to the National Cottonseed Products Association website, If we assume that only five percent of the oil in the French Cruller is from cottonseed, then the amount of CPFA's would be somewhere from 10 to 20 milligrams. The number could be higher or lower because we do not know how much cottonseed oil is in the doughnut.

"Cottonseed oil has been a part of the American diet for well over a century. Until the 1940's, it was the major vegetable oil produced in the United States. Now, with annual production averaging more than 1 billion pounds, **Cottonseed oil** ranks third in volume behind soybean and corn oil representing about 5-6% of the total domestic fat and oil supply. . . As a salad oil, it is used in mayonnaise, salad dressings, sauces, and marinades. As cooking oil, it is used for frying in both commercial and home cooking. As a shortening or margarine, it is ideal for baked goods and cake icings."

Doughnuts are just one example of foods fried in cottonseed oil. Salad dressings often contain pure cottonseed oil. Some brands of potato chips use pure cottonseed oil.[41] Many other foods contain cottonseed oil. Check the labels! At Passover time, many Jewish households use pure cottonseed oil for cooking, because of religious restrictions on certain grains. According to the National Cottonseed Products Association, as recently as July 2012, "Cottonseed oil can be found as an ingredient in many food products and is available on the grocery shelf only in limited areas." In addition, according to the National Cottonseed Products Association, "Cottonseed oil is primarily used in the U.S. as a salad or cooking oil. About 56% is consumed in that category while about 36% goes into baking and frying fats, and a small amount into margarine and other uses."[42]

What about dairy products? The amount of CPFA's in milk has been measured. Hawkins et. al., (1985) measured CPFA in milk from dairy cows fed cottonseed. These researchers found CPFA quantity of 59.6 mg/g dairy fat in the milk, (00.00596% of the fat). This translates into the amount of CPFA's present in the milk fat of a dairy cow fed cottonseed is about 60 ppm. [43]

How does this number relate to what people actually eat? If a person ate the equivalent of 1/3 stick of butter per day, they would consume about 40 grams of fat or 2.4 milligrams of CPFA's from dairy fat. Although most people don't eat plain butter in those quantities, think about the other sources of dairy fat: milk, ice cream, cheese, cream, half and half, and other dairy products.

What about meat and fat of animals? Animals which are fed cottonseed store at least some of the CPFA's in their fat. In some studies, the percentage of CPFA's in the fat approaches the CPFA content of the diet. Roehm et. al., (1971) fed rainbow trout 100 ppm or 200 ppm CPFA's and found that the amount of CPFA in the fish fat approached the percentage in the diet, in this case, 0.1% to 0.2% of the total lipid (fat).vi Accumulation in the tissues occurred for 100 days. The CPFA's were intact in the fat. This is a higher percentage than found in the dairy fat. [44]

Rabbit studies showed that in rabbits fed CPFA at 0.25%, the amount of CPFA's in the rabbit fat approached 14%.[45]Extrapolating to beef cattle, if beef cattle eat 5% whole cottonseed, the percentage of the diet as CPFA would be 0.00012 or 0.012%. Then the percentage of CPFA's in the fat of the cattle would be at least this amount. Keep in mind that this is a conservative low estimate. In actual studies of animals such as rabbits fed CPFA's, the amount of CPFA's that remained in the fat were much higher than the amount in the dietary fat.

Extra lean ground beef can contain up to 15% fat. If we use the number of 0.012%, the fat will contain 0.012% CPFA.

The amount of CPFA in the meat would work as follows for someone eating 220 grams of beef per day or two quarter- pound hamburgers. The 220 grams of beef would contain 33 grams of fat, which would in turn contain 0.012 % CPFA or about 4 milligrams of CPFA's.

These calculations have been made to show the quantity of CPFA a person would take in on a hypothetical but average diet in the United States.

So a person eating one doughnut per day, two ¼ pound hamburgers containing extra lean ground beef, and enough dairy products to contain one third stick of butter would take in somewhere between 10-20 milligrams from the doughnut, 2.4 milligrams from the butter and 4 milligrams from the beef for a total of between 16.4 to 26.4 milligrams. 16.4 milligrams per day out of an average diet containing about 500 grams per day diet[46] would be a percentage of 0.00328% CPFA to 0.00528% by weight in the whole diet. These numbers seem small but are they? Should you care?

Now I compare for you the numbers derived above, based on the potential amount of CPFA's in the human diet, with the amount of CPFA's in the experimental diet that I used. Recall that I had five groups of experimental animals: two of the groups received whole cottonseed, which contains CPFA's. Those groups were WCS-1 and WCS-2. Recall that one animal of 13 in WCS-1 and three animals of 13 in WCS-2 developed atherosclerosis. In my study, the percentage of CPFA in the WCS 2 diet was approximately 0.0004% of the rat diet. This is much less as a percentage than the numbers we just calculated for the hypothetical human diet. The example I gave above of the person eating one doughnut, two ¼ pound hamburgers and a 1/3 stick of butter per day would be between 8.2 and 13 times the percentage in the animal diet which caused heart disease. In other words, there is more than enough CPFA to cause heart disease in people. This diet is not an unreasonable starting place for creating a comparison to an experimental diet. If we look at the percentage of fat in the diet of someone who eats the way I describe, this works out to be about 31% calories as fat.[47]

To look at this calculation a different way, a person consuming an average amount of food per day would need to take in about 36 grams of dairy fat per day to eat the same percentage of CPFA as WCS-2 rats. This is the amount in approximately 1/3 of a stick of butter and less than the amount in one doughnut per day.

Practical Considerations for You

This is the end of the math. Let us review. I calculated the amount of both gossypol and CPFA that are present in the normal human diet. I calculated approximately what percentage of the diet this was, and created an animal feed to contain these amounts. There are several other toxins in cottonseed that have not been studied as much as gossypol and CPFA, but they are also present in this experimental diet because I used whole cottonseed.

Even at these low amounts, the rats developed Alzheimer's and other major diseases. The implications for people are enormous. Even with gossypol level of approximately the human diet, and a CPFA level at approximately an eighth of the human diet, rats developed Alzheimer's, heart disease, and bleeding in the brain.

This means that every time you eat a product containing CPFA, cottonseed or gossypol, whether in cottonseed oil, or in meat, fish or dairy products from an animal that has been fed cottonseed, you are increasing your risk of heart disease, Alzheimer's, and other major life threatening problems. If I were in your position, regardless of whether additional scientific studies are ever done, I would stop eating cottonseed.

Should older people also avoid cottonseed, or has the damage already been done?

You might say that this is pretty obvious for young people. You may wonder, however, is stopping cottonseed later in life is worth it, or has all of the damage been done? If so, then why bother changing eating habits?

I can't answer that question for certain. Based on the animal studies, humans may have a maximum tolerance level for cottonseed over the course of a lifetime, just as animals do. In animals, as I explained earlier, scientists and farmers know that they can only feed an animal a certain amount of cottonseed before the cottonseed toxins kill the animal. Nobody has done these studies on humans, so we must extrapolate from the known data. More research needs to be done.

However, the results of my experiment help us with this question. Bleeding, atherosclerosis, and Alzheimer's did not develop until the rats were at least two years old or older. For a rat, this is very late in life. We did not find these problems in younger rats. Experimental results show that the rats had to eat cottonseed for most of their life to develop some or all of these problems. This time frame indicates that something is occurring as the rats age. Either some effect of the cottonseed is being stored up as the rats become older, or the cottonseed toxins are accumulating and only when a threshold amount has been reached do problems develop.

In the Alzheimer's lesions seen in several of the older WCS-2 rats (rats fed the larger amounts of whole cottonseed), we found several examples of fields of neurofibrillary tangles. "Fields" means that we found many neurofibrillary tangles within a small area, not just one or two scattered neurofibrillary tangles in the whole brain. This finding is generally unusual in the brains of people who have died from Alzheimer's. In the brains of those people, neurofibrillary tangles are usually single, distributed randomly, and can be hard to find.

Why might we have found fields of neurofibrillary tangles? The reason is likely that when a critical amount of cottonseed toxin is present, the neurofibrillary tangles form and are easily visible. Given that the rats are all very similar and are eating the same diet, then the process of accumulation in the brain is occurring, leading to more lesions forming at the same time in close proximity. From other studies, scientists know that gossypol accumulates in the brains of animals. In pigs, for example, scientists have found about 8 ppm in the brain tissues of pigs which have been fed normal amounts of cottonseed. Gossypol is clearly entering the brains of animals. There is no evidence that the gossypol acts any differently in human beings.

The data from my experiment supports this conclusion. Recall that I fed one group of rats only 1 ppm of cottonseed toxins (WCS-1), and another group approximately ten times that amount (WCS-2). While we found fields of neurofibrillary tangles for the rats fed the higher concentration of toxins, we found results more comparable to human findings for the other rats. In the WCS-I rats, I found scattered neurofibrillary tangles, in numbers closer to the amount that are typically found in adults with Alzheimer's. Thus, it appears that the greater the concentration of cottonseed toxins, the more neurofibrillary tangles there are.

Why is this information important to understand? A critical amount of accumulation of cottonseed toxin may be necessary for Alzheimer's lesions to form. If we can stop the process of accumulation before this critical level is reached, perhaps the person will not develop Alzheimer's. So even for an older person, not eating cottonseed would be worthwhile.

These findings mean that eating the amount of cottonseed toxin in the current common human diet in the United States poses a major risk for developing Alzheimer's Disease and other problems.

We observed the same types of findings for atherosclerosis, the heart disease that is caused by CPFA's. In this study, we found atherosclerosis, including one very severe lesion, in the rats fed the WCS-2 diet. Three of 13 rats developed atherosclerosis and one rat out of 13 WCS-1 rats developed atherosclerosis. As I explained above, the amount of CPFA was only about an eighth of the amount in the human diet. Our study showed that eating small amounts of CPFA from whole cottonseed over a rat lifetime, caused atherosclerosis. Human beings conservatively eat, on average, about 8 to 13 times the amount of CPFA's that I used in my studies. A summary of calculations shows that a person eating one doughnut, two ¼ pound hamburgers and 1/3 stick of butter per day would take in 8 to 13 times the amount of CPFA's that the WCS 2 rats ate (which caused 3 of 13 to develop atherosclerosis). Recall that rats do not normally develop atherosclerosis, so these findings are significant.

Should you worry about this?

Again, the answer is "yes!"

There are plenty of CPFA's in the human diet to cause major heart disease. We take in cottonseed toxins in our food which cause increased cholesterol and heart disease. There are enough studies together with our experiment to show that anyone concerned about cholesterol and heart disease should worry about CPFA intake at current levels in the diet.

Should these findings convince you that cottonseed in your food is a problem? Yes. The costs of controlling one's diet are fairly low. Inconvenience in a modern world is a small price to pay for good health. Remember, cottonseed is not even a food for people. It is a product that was created as a convenience for the cottonseed industry to be able to dispose of and profit from. Cottonseed was not developed for human health or nutrition.

Until someone or some agency decides to research this problem, which I explain later is unlikely to happen, cottonseed will remain in the food supply.

Ultimately, the choice is yours. Fortunately, you have the power to make the right choice.

How to eliminate cottonseed toxins from your diet

I've told you that eliminating cottonseed from your diet is critical for you to avoid the risk of major health problems.

The question now is, how? This question is considered in the next chapter.

CHAPTER 6

HOW TO AVOID COTTONSEED IN YOUR FOOD

If you decide that, based on the research presented here, you would like to avoid cottonseed, how would you go about doing so? Cottonseed poisons are found in dairy products, in all commercially raised meat, in all farm fed fish and in chicken and turkey. The only concentrated protein food which does not have cottonseed poisons are eggs. You also get toxins from cottonseed oil, which is pressed from whole cottonseed. The poison, the cyclopropenoid fatty acids is found primarily in the oil. People eat cottonseed oil directly in foods such as salad dressings and other prepared foods.

The only way to protect yourself is to avoid these foods. Start by avoiding cottonseed oil. Anytime you see cottonseed oil on a label, you should avoid that food. Cottonseed oil is used heavily commercially, so unless one can read a label, one should avoid foods which are fried or contain commercial oils. Often in restaurants, one cannot see how the food is prepared. Then one has to avoid the fried foods there. Cheaper baked goods, such as donuts often are prepared using cottonseed oil. Many salad dressing and sauces have cottonseed oil. I suggest avoiding all these foods.

The harder problem is how to avoid cottonseed toxins which are found in beef, pork, poultry and dairy products. Dairy and beef cattle are fed whole cottonseed.[48] Whole cottonseed contains all the cottonseed toxins and all could pass through into beef and into dairy products. Cottonseed meal is fed to poultry, pigs and farm fed fish. Cottonseed meal contains a little cottonseed oil and will contain most of the other cottonseed toxins. Again all the toxins in the meal could pass on to you through the eating of fish, poultry and pork. Avoiding cottonseed toxins means avoiding all dairy products, all meat, fish and poultry. Complete avoidance is very difficult. However, if you can decrease your intake of these products, then you will decrease your total accumulation of cottonseed toxins and you will be less likely to develop cottonseed related disorders as you become older.

There are two ways to make this changeover easier. The first is to eat more eggs. Eggs contain no cottonseed and are the healthiest form of concentrated animal protein to consume. Second, I suggest eating more rice and beans. Protein foods such as meat, contain 4 kilocalories per gram of food. Rice also contains 4 kilocalories per gram. Most people eat more protein than they need and rice can be substituted for meat. The best way to substitute for the fat in meat is to put on a vegetable oil such as safflower or soy oil onto rice. Rice has some protein as well but less than meat. Third, grass fed beef contains no cottonseed but it is more expensive than regular beef. What about organic chicken? The definition of organic means raising chickens without antibiotics in clean environments and feeding the chickens only organic feed. Is there organic cottonseed? Yes, there is. I don't think you are safe by buying organic chickens. I suspect that there is less cottonseed in organic chickens because they taste better than regular chicken but I do not think you are assured of avoiding cottonseed by eating organic chicken.

This is what I do. I eat eggs. I eat very little commercial butter. I prefer butter which is from pasture fed cows. I eat beans and rice, vegetables and fruit, and potatoes. I eat safflower oil. I eat whole wheat and oatmeal. I eat grass feed beef. I eat ocean caught fish.

One other suggestion to the problem of eating less meat and chicken is as follows. To eat some meat, I have suggested in the past eating veal. This is because there is less time for the cottonseed toxins to accumulate in the calf so veal is safer. So is lamb for the same reason. In addition, in my life I have had to be concerned with another problem called Candida albicans, an intestinal yeast which is responsible for much illness. This is also a problem which is addressed through dietary change. We had to write cookbooks for people who had to deal with this problem. As we wrote these cookbooks, we knew about cottonseed. Most of the recipes are fine for people who want to avoid cottonseed but there are a few meat containing recipes in these books. These books are *Feast Without Yeast* and *Extraordinary Foods for the Everyday Kitchen*.

I think if you cut your intake of cottonseed, you will do better, even if you do not eliminate it completely. Even I eat a little bit of organic kosher chicken.

CHAPTER 7

FUTURE DIRECTIONS: HYPOTHESES ABOUT THE MECHANISMS IN COTTONSEED POISONING

The problems that cottonseed causes have been presented in earlier chapters. Nobody really knows exactly how these problems occur. Nobody is currently researching the toxicity of cottonseed to humans publicly. The main medical research community is not currently concerned about the problems that cottonseed causes—or rather, they are concerned about the problems themselves, such as Alzheimer's, but they are not interested in researching whether cottonseed could be the cause. This lack of concern means that research on cottonseed is not currently incorporated in a clear direction for research into today's medical problems.

Why is this a problem? This is a problem because, if the main medical community is not interested in researching cottonseed and the problems it causes, the research is almost impossible to perform. However, the research needs to be done. So I am committed to doing this if funding is available.

This chapter is about what researchers could do if there were proper funding under the right circumstances.

In this chapter, I will present hypotheses about how cottonseed might cause the problems that have been observed. I will also present suggestions for future research, because I hope that other researchers will be interested enough in solving basic human health problems to explore these issues further.

In the next chapter, I discuss whether such research is likely to be done, given the enormous structural pressures on not doing the proposed type of research. I do this in the hope that the main research community will recognize these barriers and will then help surmount them. Only then will we truly have answers to the questions I have raised.

Hypotheses

In scientific research, we discuss mechanisms of how toxins may cause medical issues. Such thoughts and discussions concern the manner or mechanism in which toxins act upon biological structures and processes that result in the medical problems one sees

When I discuss cottonseed toxicity mechanisms, I look at the problems that result from feeding cottonseed. For example, in several studies, animals fed cottonseed bled abnormally. The question is how does cottonseed interact with the body's structures and processes such that bleeding results? Understanding such mechanisms may help us understand both bleeding and help us predict whether cottonseed may cause other problems besides bleeding. Scientists can then do further research on whether cottonseed causes different or additional health problems.

I will now present my hypotheses about mechanisms, or the way in which cottonseed toxins cause bleeding, clotting, aneurysms and heart disease. All of these issues need further research.

Mechanisms of abnormal bleeding

One of the major effects in animals of consuming cottonseed toxins is that the toxins cause unnatural and extensive bleeding.

Such bleeding in turn can cause death or stroke. As I described earlier, other scientists saw bleeding as an effect of cottonseed toxins. They found this result in four different studies.[49] Like these other scientists, we discovered major bleeding episodes in the animals in our research study. One result of extensive bleeding is an animal's early death.

We do not know from this finding, whether bleeding to death was the only problem that cottonseed caused, or whether the cottonseed toxins also affected other tissues and organs in the body, contributing to the animal's death. The bleeding is simply easiest to observe.

So now, the question: why might cottonseed toxins cause bleeding?

Bleeding results when blood does not clot properly. The blood clotting system depends on a number of proteins. Normally these proteins simply float around in the bloodstream. They are all separate from one another in the blood. An opening in a blood vessel wall signals these proteins to come together to form a clot, which is a quick structure that plugs the hole in the blood vessel wall. The whole system works in a coordinated sequential fashion.

When the blood vessel wall develops a hole, the body sends out signals to the blood clotting proteins to go into this cascading effect. The signals cause one blood clotting protein to attach to the leak, and then another and another until they build up a structure which plugs the hole. I think of this as a structure like an inverted pyramid. One protein starts the process. Then others build on it in an expanding structure. The entire system depends on having proteins that are the correct structure and are able to work together and communicate with each other. The proteins need to find the correct places to attach on each other. If something happens to cause these proteins to be unable to communicate with each other, or the structures don't fit together properly because of abnormalities in the protein structures, the system will fail and the body will be unable to form clots properly. Then a hole or tear in a blood vessel cannot be repaired and the result is uncontrolled bleeding.

What could cause problems in the proteins' ability to communicate with each other?

Recall that two things need to occur for successful clotting, proper communication and proper structure. A defect in either would inhibit clotting. Thus, one of the possibilities for how cottonseed interferes with clotting and leads to uncontrolled bleeding is that the proteins become deformed because a different substance has attached itself to a protein, changing its structure.

Let us look at what we know from past studies. In a study on the effect of gossypol on digestive enzymes, scientists found that the cottonseed toxin gossypol binds, or attaches, to one of the body's essential proteins, a digestive enzyme.[50] Gossypol binding renders this enzyme inactive. Enzymes have an active site, or place, where other chemicals fit with that enzyme like puzzle pieces. This active site can work on or modify these chemicals. In the case of this digestive enzyme (trypsin), the digestive enzyme binds a piece of protein from food in the gut and cuts it into several smaller pieces. To picture this in your mind, imagine that in a normal pair of scissors, the two blades come together around a piece of paper and cut it. However, if the scissors has a bent blade, even if the paper comes between the two blades and the two blades come together, they will not slice the paper because one of the blades is bent. Or imagine instead that one of the handles of the scissors is broke. The blades are there but they cannot move

When gossypol is present and binds to this particular digestive enzyme (trypsin), it is like bending the blade on the scissors. The structure of the digestive enzyme changes so that the digestive enzyme cannot cut the piece of the protein. In other words, the enzyme doesn't work.

Extrapolating from this finding, we can hypothesize that gossypol may bind to essential clotting proteins a similar way that it can bind to digestive enzymes. This binding would cause the protein to be deactivated or deformed. Then the clotting proteins will not bind properly and will not form a proper solid structure for clotting. Then the bleeding will continue. This explains the excessive bleeding observed in experimental animals which were fed the cottonseed poison gossypol.

Excessive bleeding is also more likely if the blood vessel walls are weak. For the same reasons discussed above, I hypothesize that gossypol makes the blood vessel walls weaker, which means they are more likely to break under stress. If gossypol binds to and deforms the proteins, then structures comprised of these proteins will be weaker because the proteins won't connect properly. By binding to the proteins making up blood vessels, gossypol could weaken the blood vessel walls. Weaker walls are more likely to break.

Think about the problem in this way: blood vessel walls are like brick walls, with the proteins as bricks. If a brick mason is trying to build a wall, he or she will have an easier time if all of the bricks are the same shape and size. What happens when every once in awhile, a brick is an odd shape or has something strange attached, like a stone or a piece of metal that shouldn't be there? The structure will be weaker, even if the mason is skilled enough to use these odd pieces of brick. Blood vessel walls are similar. The body engages in systems of continuous growth and change. Like other structures in the body, blood vessel walls are constantly being repaired, made, and expanded. If the body is trying to build and repair blood vessel walls with deformed proteins, the walls will not be structurally sound. The occasional deformed protein probably will not matter, because the body can avoid using it. But the more deformed proteins that are present in the body, the more the body will have to use these proteins, resulting in weaker structure in blood vessel walls. Weak blood vessel walls make holes in the blood vessel walls more likely. Once blood vessel walls rupture, the bleeding will continue because the blood will not clot as quickly as it should.

I have now explained two hypotheses about how gossypol could work to deform proteins in blood clotting and in blood vessel wall repair. If either or both of these hypotheses prove correct after experimentation, the mechanism involved in gossypol poisoning will be explained and we will know how and why gossypol causes excessive bleeding.

Mechanisms of abnormal clotting

The second problem relating to blood, ironically, is too much clotting in the wrong places. Recall that I discussed earlier that several studies show that the cottonseed toxin gossypol causes animals to develop spontaneous blood clots in their hearts.[51] In humans, spontaneous clots cause heart attacks and strokes. One possible cause of blood clotting in the wrong places could be similar to the mechanisms that cause excessive bleeding. Toxins attaching themselves to active sites on clotting proteins could deform or inhibit the proteins in such a way that the proteins start clotting spontaneously, leading to a clot in the wrong place, or floating in the bloodstream. Floating solid clots in the bloodstream can enter the heart or brain arteries and can lead to heart attacks and strokes.

Let me explain. The blood clotting proteins or factors normally float in the bloodstream, all separate from each other, waiting for something to happen that requires clotting. They float in such a shape that their main binding sites are not exposed to other proteins. Think of this as a long coiled strand that when unfurled, will have sites on it on which blood clotting proteins can attach to make a multi-dimensional tower. In the normal state, the long strand is curled up on itself protecting those binding sites so clotting proteins don't bind at the wrong times.

However, we know that gossypol attaches to enzymes, which are proteins. If gossypol binds to one or more of the blood clotting proteins in such a way that it signals that protein to unfurl and expose its binding sites, then other blood clotting proteins will attach to the sites, and send the cascading clotting mechanism into action to make a larger structure where no injury is present. This would result in an abnormal clot.

Gossypol may cause aortic aneurysms

I have just explained hypotheses about the mechanisms underlying two major problems in the blood, abnormal bleeding and abnormal clotting. However, clotting and bleeding problems are not isolated problems in the blood. Similar mechanisms may underlie many other problems.

A person is living, breathing, changing and evolving. When the body has problems with bleeding and clotting, the body most likely will have more problems. Blood carries oxygen to other parts of the body, and removes waste. In addition, the same problems affecting the clotting proteins may also affect other proteins throughout the body. If those other proteins are deformed or inactivated, other bodily systems will be at risk. In other words, cottonseed toxins may put any or all tissues at risk of not functioning at full potential. As I stated earlier, more research is needed to determine exactly how these problems occur, and what can be done about them.

A specific example of tissues at risk may be found in the causes of aortic aneurysms. In our study, we found an aortic aneurysm in a rat fed the higher dose of gossypol. No published paper has previously reported a finding of aortic aneurysms in animals. While this is only one animal, this finding is still significant. The animal that developed the aneurysm had been fed a diet containing ten times the amount of gossypol that would normally be found in the diet.

An aortic aneurysm is massive bleeding from the aorta, which is the major blood vessel leading from the heart. This problem occurs commonly in older human beings. Aortic aneurysms in people are devastating, often causing death. Scientists do not fully understand what causes them. Aneurysms start with weak blood vessel walls, which become thinner and, keep on expanding, thinning and weakening at the same time.

A possible mechanism explaining the aortic aneurysm could be that gossypol binds to the proteins in the blood vessel walls, weakening the walls. This would start the aneurysm process.

Mechanisms of how cottonseed toxins cause heart failure

I have discussed possible mechanisms for three problems that we know cottonseed toxins cause: excessive bleeding, clotting in the wrong places and aortic aneurysms. A fourth finding is on a different path, heart failure. Heart failure, and heart attacks, are both life-threatening and common in people.

Scientists have observed heart failure in cottonseed-fed animals.[52] This is a regular finding. Nobody knows all of the causes of heart failure. However, heart failure can occur if the heart muscle becomes weak, or does not receive enough oxygen. As described previously, we know that the cottonseed toxin gossypol binds randomly to proteins. Gossypol binding to proteins can change the shape of the proteins, causing them to be deformed and not work properly. Proteins make up the basic structures of the body, from cells to tissues to organs. Deformed

proteins, like deformed bricks, will cause the resulting structures to be weaker.

The heart, like other structures, is constantly changing and
evolving, breaking down and being repaired. This is a normal part
of life. If the proteins repairing the heart are deformed, some heart
cells could become structurally imperfect. The heart could then
have trouble continuing to beat and could fail. Cottonseed toxins
may weaken the heart muscle, making it wear out earlier than it
should. Again, this is an area for further research.

Mechanisms of how cottonseed toxins cause Atherosclerosis

A second area of heart health is atherosclerosis, which is related
to high cholesterol but is not totally the same. In my study, several
animals had atherosclerosis. Other scientists have also found atherosclerosis in animals fed cottonseed toxins. [53]

Cholesterol in the blood is free floating. Atherosclerosis is a disease that develops when the cholesterol gets stuck inside the arterial
walls, causing a buildup of cholesterol and a resulting narrowing of
the arteries. Doctors want their patients to control their cholesterol
to prevent excessive buildup, because too much cholesterol can narrow the arteries which cuts off or slows blood supply to the heart.
You probably have known someone who has had to undergo surgery
for bypassing blocked arteries.

In an earlier chapter we discussed how cottonseed toxins cause
increased cholesterol. [54]

The question is how does cottonseed toxin cause atherosclerosis? The problem of atherosclerosis is cholesterol deposition
occurring in the wrong places, the artery walls. Nobody knows
how this process starts. It is possible that similar mechanisms to

those discussed above relating to excessive clotting and excessive bleeding are underway in cholesterol deposition in arteries.

We do know that the inside lining of the arteries is in a natural state very smooth. The arteries are made of proteins. Whenever there is a break in an artery wall, the clotting mechanism is thrown into action, as it is for any other blood vessel. As I explained above, this mechanism, when operating normally, plugs the break and begins the repair process. If the artery walls are repaired with deformed proteins, they might not be as smooth as they should be. In addition, the artery walls could become "hard" or less flexible, that is, less elastic and more rigid over time. Arteries are under pressure, because the heart pumps blood through the arteries with sufficient pressure to keep it circulating throughout the body. Rigid walls are more likely to break or rupture under pressure. Over time the breaks may become bigger and harder to fix quickly, allowing blood to enter the space under the cells lining the artery. The blood contains cholesterol and some of the cholesterol may be left behind in the crack in the blood vessel wall. Gossypol also may bind to cholesterol. Gossypol could both bind to the damaged blood vessel wall and to the cholesterol, starting the atherosclerotic plaque. No one knows the process which begins the atherosclerotic deposition of cholesterol. The ideas advanced in this paragraph must be researched further. [55]

Mechanisms of how cottonseed toxins cause genetic mutations

There is yet one more major possibility of damage that scientists should research, that is, the foundation of our entire life structure, our genes in the form of DNA. A pair of Swedish researchers reported in 1984 that gossypol induced DNA strand breaks and unusual exchange of genetic material across chromosomes in human cells.[56] These effects result in genetic mutations. I do not know of any other food which contains "genotoxic" elements. Gossypol is a primary candidate for causing any problem which results from DNA mutations which accumulate over time.

One such condition seems to be autism. Older men are more likely to father children with autism. This is thought to be due to the accumulation of "spontaneous" genetic mutations over time. But might these "spontaneous" genetic mutations really come from the accumulation of gossypol and its effects over time? Perhaps gossypol is the cause of these mutations. Thus gossypol may be one factor causing an increase in the rate of autism diagnosis.[57]

Gossypol is known to damage DNA. There is a negative impact of cottonseed on male fertility and female cows cannot be fed too much cottonseed or they will not produce calves. No one knows whether our bodies can protect and preserve our DNA from damage over a lifetime of gossypol induced DNA changes and mutations, both in reproductive and in other body cells. These questions are in desperate need of research.

Further Research

What I have suggested here are hypotheses about the ways by which cottonseed toxins cause the damage that we see in the research lab and on the farm. Although we don't completely understand the exact mechanisms right now, I hope that further research will give us more information. I have suggested some future research paths that may be productive, based on the results of the studies done thus far.

But is such future research likely to happen? I would like to think that it is. I suspect, however, that such research may be a long time in coming. The priorities of the research world are not the same and will be considered in the next chapter.

CHAPTER 8

OVERCOMING BARRIERS FOR CHANGE

In earlier chapters, I have shown you why eating cottonseed is bad for you. I hope that I have accomplished my goal of helping you understand the scientific studies. I also showed you how pervasive cottonseed is in our modern diets, and how feeding cottonseed to animals is a major part of the agricultural economy.

I have also discussed the possible reasons why cottonseed toxins gossypol and cyclopropenoid fatty acids (CPFA's) cause the observed problems. I have suggested avenues for further research to ensure the safety of our food supply and ultimately, our health.

I would like to think that the scientific merit of doing further studies on cottonseed toxins would prompt other researchers to jump onboard and continue the research to protect our health. However, I am skeptical that this will happen anytime soon without major structural changes in the way research is funded and conducted. In order to understand the structural barriers in the research world that must be overcome, you need to know something about the economics of cottonseed production and research.

Barriers to change: The economics and politics of cottonseed research

Why has cottonseed become such a pervasive part of our diet? Why does cottonseed slowly poison us? The answer to this question lies partly in economic incentives and partly on understanding the world of scientific research. Economic incentives are relatively easy to see. The cotton industry produces seeds, which can be a huge problem unless farmers can get rid of them. That was the beginning of the use of cottonseed as animal feed. Now cottonseed is a large part of the agricultural economy. It is a cheap source of animal feed, and a large source of inexpensive cooking oil and other ingredients in manufactured food products. So, there is little economic incentive to eliminate this cheap and readily available source of feed. Cotton is a heavily subsidized agricultural commodity. The more cotton that is grown, the more cottonseed there is. Because it is cheap, it is fed as much as possible.

The research community has both been funded by and supported by the cottonseed industry. Cottonseed is part of the agricultural system and is well established in part because of all the research that scientists have done to determine the levels of cottonseed that farmers could "safely" feed to animals. Thus, the research has been aimed at making cottonseed a usable feed. The research was not directed at making cottonseed a safe source of feed for humans, in any way.

At any time since 1915, the wisdom of allowing cottonseed toxins to enter human food could have been questioned. However, this question has never been asked in any public way. Why?

The people who performed this research owed their jobs to cottonseed. The question of whether cottonseed in the food chain was safe in the long run was not their concern. The cottonseed producers did not fund the question, the scientists did not study the question, and people just generally assumed that if the cottonseed didn't kill the animals directly, it was OK.

Should these researchers have asked whether the research was a good idea for the national health of Americans in the future. They could have (a) continued the research because that is what they were paid to do; or (b) decided not to do the research because maybe putting all that poison into the human food supply was not such a great idea. An individual researcher could have said maybe all that poison was not such a great idea but who wants to tackle the entire cottonseed industry?

For an individual researcher to have raised such questions would have been difficult for a number of reasons. First, the researcher wanted to continue to work. But second, almost all of these researchers were agricultural people who were not expected to know about human medicine and medical problems. Except for excessive bleeding, there was no research showing direct links in those years. In 1915, Alzheimer's was barely being described. Perhaps they could have asked a medical colleague about correlations to human medical problems but I think that would have been about all.

What about the system of research?

As we noted earlier, "the problem of cottonseed injury" was noted back in the 1800's. The toxic effects of gossypol were documented as early as 1915 by Withers and Carruth. I described their study in which they fed cottonseed to rabbits, which killed the rabbits. Withers and Carruth concluded that "the feeding experiments show that gossypol is very poisonous." Every subsequent researcher would have been familiar with this study. Withers and Carruth also stated that the value of the cottonseed crop at that time was $53 million. The citing of this figure in an academic paper simply shows that money was important.

Although we like to think that political and economic considerations do not control research, let's examine the question further.

Did researchers after 1915 in any way attempt to do research to determine whether the extremely poisonous cottonseed toxin was safe for people? Not in any reported studies. Their research was limited to making cottonseed safe for the animals. The cottonseed farmers formed an association, still in existence today, to promote research into cottonseed so that it could be used as part of animal feed. They convinced the United States Department of Agriculture (USDA) to sponsor research into making cottonseed a possible food for animals. Many of the studies came from USDA labs. Withers and Carruth were in a USDA lab. If the cottonseed farmers had not formed such an association and funded research on cottonseed, and if the USDA had not supported the research, it is unlikely that feeding cottonseed to animals would have continued, because the cottonseed was killing the animals.

Both University labs and USDA labs researched exactly how much cottonseed could be fed to animals and fish without killing them. There were programs to determine how to process the cottonseed to remove some of the poison, enabling more cottonseed to be fed to animals. These research projects were very active at least from the 1920's to the 1960's. There were major scientific meetings devoted to sharing information about how to make cottonseed a viable food for farm animals.

The whole goal of the research was to determine how much cottonseed could be fed to the animals and allow them to grow. By the 1960's, cottonseed was well established as part of the agriculture system. Pigs and chicken were fed cottonseed routinely. Initially not so much was fed to beef and dairy cattle because they could eat cheaper foods such as hay. With dairy cows there was concern about how much could be fed and the animals still have reproductive function, but these amounts were determined. Cottonseed then became a major part of cattle feed.

The long term health of people is not mentioned in any research study since 1915 except for one which will be discussed below. Any researcher who might have thought about the ethics of feeding toxic cottonseed to animals would have been out of a job. If that researcher questioned the wisdom of putting all that cottonseed poison into animals which human beings would then eat, their research money would have dried up. No one was going to be paid for considering the toxicology of the levels of cottonseed found in meat. No one considered it their responsibility. The scientists also were not trained in toxicology or medicine. They did not have the tools to consider possible disorders which might be caused by eating cottonseed at the levels found in meat.

The economics of the cottonseed industry has controlled research on cottonseed to date. Is it any wonder that the safety of cottonseed in the human diet has never been studied? Was all this research ethical? This is a free country. People can organize and spend their money as they wish. Should there have been research on cottonseed with the goal to protect the health of people and if so, why was there not such research?

Scientists then, as now, should have a third choice (c), to research the safety of cottonseed toxins in the modern human diet. Creating a choice (c) will require new funding that is independent of the cottonseed industry and probably the USDA. The purpose of the research would be to determine whether eating cottonseed regularly for periods of time is safe for people.

Only two scientists to date, myself and a veterinarian named S. Morgan, DVM, in 1988,[58] have even raised the question of whether cottonseed is safe to eat in the long run. There is no published study showing that eating food containing cottonseed toxins is safe for people. I repeat, we have multiple studies showing that cottonseed is toxic to animals and causes sterility in male animals, and nobody has ever shown the opposite—that cottonseed is safe for consumption. We only know that farmers can feed a certain amount to their livestock without destroying them.

The continued research support for feeding cottonseed is one of the worst and most costly decisions that ever occurred in American history. As I have shown in my study, and as has been shown as early as 1915, feeding cottonseed causes mortal problems for animals, and is retained in the meat and fat of animals that people eat. As I have shown throughout this book, the cottonseed toxins that animals eat lead to major heart problems, stroke, and Alzheimer's.

So, let us review: the economics of the cottonseed industry have shaped the research on cottonseed toxins. The research leads people to assume that because cottonseed is in our food, it is safe. Nobody has researched whether eating cottonseed toxins in our food supply is safe over the long term.

Today, I hope that a leader in research will emerge who will care about the long term health of the population, particularly given the enormous costs of Alzheimer's and other diseases. Economic and special interests should not govern scientific research.

Unfortunately, such research is not likely to be funded or conducted. That is because of an entirely different problem in the research world: the inherent structure of biomedical research.

Barriers to change: The structure of biomedical research

Even apart from economic concerns, even assuming that a researcher wanted to look into the long term safety of cottonseed, the structure of medical and scientific research inhibits this type of work. The way biomedical research works at the very least hinders the type of long-term, large-scale research projects that need to be conducted for evaluating the safety of cottonseed toxins.

Let us look at how medical research works.

Medical research is conducted in university or medical school laboratories. The labs are headed by scientist faculty members. Labs are organized into basic disciplines, such as biochemistry, genetics, or neurosciences. Scientists within labs try to focus their questions within their own disciplines. Geneticists ask questions about genetics. Neurologists ask questions about neurology.

The scientists depend on grants for their life blood. Universities do not fully fund labs. If you talk to any researcher, that person is always in the process of writing a grant, thinking about writing a grant, completing writing a grant, or waiting for a decision on a grant, or all of the above. These grants fund the laboratory, including equipment and chemicals, and a major part of salaries and fellowships. These scientists frequently have students working for them, usually graduate students or post-doctoral fellows, who must be funded and who must produce publishable results. Grants are usually short term, at most a few years, and must generate publishable results or future grants will not be funded. Research fellows and students also have time limits. They cannot study forever. They need to complete their studies in a few months or years, then look for jobs in research doing—you guessed it, writing grants.

With this structure, an ideal study can be done in three to six months which generates results which can then be written up the results for a publication. The publication process also takes time. Meanwhile, the lab would be doing other studies. The results of this research would then be used by the graduate student to earn a Ph.D. or by the post-doctoral fellow to obtain funding and a job. The study could not be too complex or too long, because it would take too long to complete. Usually, the focus of the study would be entirely within one discipline such as genetics or biochemistry, because then everyone within the discipline could read it and could see that the research should be funded further. A single-focused lab can study a gene to see if it is important or not. The research would be in an area deemed "relevant and important," because otherwise, who would fund it?

This model builds on current knowledge and extends the research a little further so that the outcome is more or less predictable, but not so far that the research is risky and may not show anything. Even then, not everything is going to work, but scientists try to maximize the probability that an experiment will be successful. Finally, studies should form the basis for future studies and grants which bring money into the university.

Perhaps more important for a university, such research should not be political and should not be in opposition to some other large organization's agenda.

The agricultural studies done on cottonseed toxins met most of those criteria. The studies were short term; they were considered relevant and important in their day and the outcomes were predictable. The cottonseed studies brought cottonseed money into the universities. Therefore, such studies were done in university and USDA laboratories. No large organization was upset or opposed to this research. Once the research determined how to use cottonseed without killing the animals involved, most of the research stopped because the goal had been accomplished.

Nothing is wrong with this research model for myriad areas of medical research. Certainly, doctors and scientists have made extraordinary discoveries using this structure of research. The current hot topics are stem cells, developing new drugs and on identifying genes which may be involved in disease processes.

Unfortunately, these topics do not include long term effects of dietary toxins.

I am not suggesting or advocating changing the entire structure of medical research. I am only suggesting that the structure may prevent the discovery of other problems and solutions. A new model needs to be developed to research the long term impact of cottonseed toxicity.

In the current research world, anything that is outside the existing model cannot be done easily. If a study takes too long, and would generate results only after a long period of time, that study is unlikely to be funded. If a study challenges traditional beliefs, the study is unlikely to be funded. If the study is done somehow, and produces results which challenge traditional beliefs, the study is unlikely to be published because the people reviewing studies for publication have the same focus on current knowledge within a single discipline. Thus, the studies will not likely be published, and further research will never get funded because there are no publishable results. And ironically, people will criticize the few who raise the questions about cottonseed poisoning stating that there are no published studies showing that cottonseed is toxic in the human diet. It is a vicious circle. But wait, there's more.

A useful study of a dietary poison would also involve large numbers of animals, and it would go for their lifetimes. Such studies cannot be done quickly and their outcome is not totally predictable. In addition, a useful study on the medical toxicity of cottonseed would cross disciplines. A single lab could not study a dietary poison without input from many other people and disciplines. They would need an agricultural researcher who knows about cottonseed, a toxicologist who knows about poisons, and a pathologist who can look at the effects on the body. Multi-disciplinary studies require cooperation, division of labor and funding, and different types of grants. The agencies which review funding proposals are also organized into disciplines, making it harder for a multi-disciplinary proposal to be considered. Several researchers from different disciplines would have to agree on a proposed project, and grant funders would need to fund it.

Let us look at how many different disciplines would be involved and how long the study would take to investigate a dietary cause of Alzheimer's. Alzheimer's and diet by definition cuts across several disciplines. Someone would have to know how to construct an experimental diet. The nutritionists know how to construct a diet, but they are not trained in toxicology. A toxicologist would be needed to plan how much of the poison to give and for how long. An expert in long term feeding studies would be needed to gauge the animals' progress. A veterinarian would be needed for the animals' health and to assess the effects of the diet. An expert in the brain would be needed to determine what studies to do on the brain and how to handle the brain specimens to maximize the possibility of obtaining results. A psychologist would be needed to do memory tests on the animals as they age. All these people would have to agree on the design of the study. The reality is that such a group of people would be very unlikely to come together.

If they did come together, how long would the study take? If one were to study a dietary poison that affects people, one would first have to decide which one is worth studying. One would have to decide the level of the poison to put in the experimental diet. One would need to know the amount of the poison in our food so that one could design a diet that is close to that level. Otherwise, people would not take the results seriously. The study would also take a long time, several years. People do not eat large amounts of poison over a short time (usually). Rather, they eat low levels of poison over the course of their life. The lifetime of a rat is two to three years, so that would be the minimum amount of time for the study, plus additional time to analyze the results. To approximate the effect on people, one would need to feed comparable amounts that would approximate the human accumulation over a lifetime.

Results are never guaranteed. The lab doing the study would need to be willing to take the risk of finding no results, or doing a preliminary study over the course of a few years to get preliminary results, then doing a larger study. All of this takes time. The average lab is not able to do this type of long term study because results could not be achieved quickly enough for the needs of the labs, the students, post-doctoral fellows and funding agencies.

For funding, not only would a multi-disciplinary group need to come together to do research, they would need to apply for funding. Dietary toxins are not a hot topic. In fact, the very idea that food is important in human health, and that dietary toxins cause an impact on health, is not popular. Thus, these ideas are hard to fund.

If a group of scientists did come together, which agency would fund the research? The National Institutes of Health (NIH) funds most medical research. The NIH is divided into institutes, such as the National Institute on Aging, the National Cancer Institute, and so forth. Which of these agencies would even review such a proposal, assuming that a proposal could be developed?

Let us look for at the evaluation process for funding research. This process is just as political as anything else. Research proposals go to other scientists in the same field for review. At the national level, these groups are called study sections. At foundations, there may be a review board of scientists. These scientists review proposals and assign priority scores for funding. If the proposals being submitted and the reviewers come from the same types of research areas, the proposal will most likely be looked at favorably. However, if the proposal being submitted is very different and/or challenges reviewers' basic assumptions, the reviewers are not likely to be able to assess the proposal well and are likely to reject it or give it a very low priority score. The proposal will probably not be funded. This can be true also of private research foundations. Such a study could occur in an ideal world, if someone had enough money to fund it. The National Institute on Aging, for example, could decide to fund labs to look at all possibilities for causes of Alzheimer's. That step would be revolutionary. This has not yet happened. To make this happen, someone very influential in research would need to decide that looking outside the normal research box was important.

The economic importance of cottonseed, sadly, has an impact on the research world. I wondered what happened to CPFA research showing that CPFA's caused high cholesterol in rabbits in only five weeks. The research came to an end in the 1980's. The researchers could no longer obtain grant funding. I talked with one of the researchers who had had to leave his lab and the University and start working as a toxicologist for a large company. He said there were political issues and would not say more. In five weeks of feeding CPFA to rabbits, the rabbits developed atherosclerosis and the research has to stop.

If ideas concerning food toxicity do not receive funding, scientists won't work on these issues because funding private research is too expensive. My experience taught me this lesson! We decided, through Wisconsin Institute of Nutrition, LLP, to use the profits from our books (titles given in the footnote)[59] to fund our small study. We were able to do so over the course of four years. I had to rent space, retrofit that space to be a safe research laboratory and comply with animal safety standards, obtain racks and cages for the animals, as well as obtain equipment to mix diets, pay lab assistants and a University pathologist to analyze samples, and obtain the raw materials for the study. Obtaining those materials was not easy. When I contacted the chemical company to obtain gossypol, for example, the company would not give me a customer number. They allowed me to purchase a small amount of gossypol, but would never make me a regular customer. When I tried to buy cottonseed, I had to purchase the seed through feed stores in Wisconsin and in Texas, explaining that I was feeding animals. People were very suspicious. Purchasing equipment for the laboratory was easier, but extremely expensive because all laboratory equipment seems to be priced as if someone else (the US Government) is paying. The entire study cost for animal care, rent and personnel cost over $100,000.

Once the study was completed, there is an additional problem: that is, the study must be published. The same process occurs in publication as in funding grants. If a research study is too out of bounds for current scientific thinking, it is not likely to get published no matter how meritorious, because the study cannot survive the assessments of the reviewers. Let me give you an example. Having a Ph.D. in nutrition, as well as an M.D., I have had many experiences being published as an author of scientific papers. My colleague who performed the pathology also has a Ph.D., and works at a major university. We had set up the experiment according to protocol and had performed it to the best of our resources and abilities. So I was surprised by the reception these findings received.

We submitted the findings to a number of scientific journals that dealt with nutrition, Alzheimer's, aging and general pathology. Generally, before publication, journals send out the proposed articles to reviewers if they think the topic is worthy of publication. I submitted my paper to multiple journals that should have been interested. The American Society for Nutrition (a group of professional nutrition researchers) of which I am a member, took one look at the title and returned the paper within a day, stating they were just not interested. Were they really not interested in the possible dietary causes of Alzheimer's? The American Institute of Pathology had the same response, but kept my $50 submission fee.

Most of the journals that did send the paper out to reviewers yielded interesting, if disappointing, results. Some researchers commented simply that they just didn't believe the results, no matter what the photos showed, because nobody had ever shown this before. One reviewer said that rats do not develop Alzheimer's; therefore these findings are not real. They did not, however, take into consideration that nobody has done this experiment. Another reviewer, however, thought that the findings were very exciting. Unfortunately, that person was in the minority. That reviewer was outnumbered by two others who found many things wrong in the paper and never really addressed the main ideas. The editor of this journal told me they simply did not believe the findings and would not look further at the paper.

The researchers' attitude, that if a result were real, someone should have shown it before, shows just how hard it is to publish new findings. Contrast this skepticism with the numerous studies published by agricultural scientists showing that feeding large amounts of cottonseed causes major problems in animals. The purpose of these studies is to show what the highest level of cottonseed is that animals can eat without dying. These studies have been published, and are informative. Other published studies show that cottonseed toxins are stored in animal fat. Would it not be interesting for the scientific community to learn about what happens when people eat those stored toxins?

What could be one cause of this skepticism? Generally, within the medical and scientific community, convincing scientists and doctors that diet has anything to do with disease is a challenge. My findings are unexpected, and seemingly difficult to believe because believing them would require scientists to make the link between diet and disease. A further cause for skepticism was possibly the low-tech nature of the experiment. I fed rats and made observations. My findings in this study were based on observation in a light microscope, which generally would have been very acceptable thirty years ago, because at that time, Alzheimer's was diagnosed by these same techniques. However, Alzheimer's research has become much more high tech and expensive, requiring molecular biology and genetics techniques. Scientific journals appear to prefer the high-tech approach. The slides that we produced based on real pathological findings, of neurofibrillary tangles inside brain cells, would have been sufficient thirty years ago to show that cottonseed poisons cause Alzheimer's lesions. These lesions look exactly like what has been seen under the microscope for 100 years. For anyone concerned about developing Alzheimer's in his or her lifetime, this information is extremely valuable because then at least one would know that avoiding cottonseed poisons would help in avoiding Alzheimer's.

The point is, an unknown researcher, even with a University background, a Ph.D., an MD, and several other published papers like myself, who does not receive government funding and who broaches a new topic with a new perspective, is unlikely to get published. Without publication, there can be no funding. Without funding, there is no research. So these ideas may never see the light of day.

Fortunately, the journal, *Medical Hypotheses*, a peer-reviewed journal, recognized the value of my study, and for that I am thankful.[60]

Overcoming these Barriers to Change

To review: Cottonseed growers fund the research, which states that cottonseed can be fed to animals without killing them. People may assume from this that cottonseed is safe for people, but that has never been shown. Only two researchers, I and Morgan[61] have even raised the question of whether cottonseed is safe for people. Combine this problem with the structure of medical research and the small likelihood that future research on this question will be funded. This all seems pretty hopeless and frustrating.

But there is hope. We do not know the exact extent to which cottonseed toxins contribute to the major killers and diseases in our society: stroke, heart disease, and Alzheimer's. This book has tried to show how cottonseed could be contributing to these disorders. The cost of these diseases to society is astronomical. The cottonseed industry may be profitable and very large compared with a lone researcher's voice. However, the total value of the cottonseed crop pales in comparison to the health costs of diseases such as stroke and heart disease and Alzheimer's.

I am hopeful that someone, perhaps a reader, will recognize that our society will be much better off if we stop feeding cottonseed to animals and we stop using cottonseed oil. Then our national health bill will go down and people will be healthier. Our politicians should think about it.

I have started a non-profit research foundation, Wisconsin Institute of Nutrition Research Foundation, Inc., dedicated to funding the types of research that will improve our health. You are already part of the solution by reading this book. You can go further by not eating cottonseed containing foods, and you can contribute to further research in this area by visiting our website, http://wisresearch. com/.

Your help will be so appreciated.

APPENDIX A

SUMMARIES OF SCIENTIFIC STUDIES ON COTTONSEED TOXICITY

This Appendix summarizes the actual studies on cottonseed toxicity. These studies are presented here for readers who want greater detail. As the reader reviews the studies, contrast them in your mind with the Cottonseed Producers Association's statements that cottonseed is perfectly safe.

I described earlier in the book how all of these studies used high levels of cottonseed toxin to produce acute results. Such studies tell other researchers what to look for and give an idea of the expectations of a longer term toxicity study using lower amounts of the toxins. These studies also give an idea of the general level of toxicity.

General toxicity and gossypol

1. *Withers and Carruth: toxicity of cottonseed in pigs and rabbits*[62]

Withers and Carruth are the researchers who created the foundation for further research on cottonseed. They conducted several experiments, published in 1915, leading them to be the first to conclude that cottonseed is toxic. Every cottonseed researcher after this 1915 study read this paper. What is particularly noteworthy in this first paper is not only that Withers and Carruth showed that in pigs, rabbits and rats cottonseed was highly toxic, but that these researchers gave extremely vivid descriptions of their pathological findings.

The first experiment involved feeding pigs fed a ration containing cottonseed meal at 1% of their body weight. The pigs died within weeks.

Withers and Carruth followed this line of research with several experiments on rabbits. They sought to feed rabbits more refined cottonseed toxin. The first several experiments used extracts that contained gossypol, but also contained other cottonseed poisons. Withers and Carruth first noted that rabbits will not eat cottonseed meal. They had to mix the cottonseed in molasses. Then the rabbits would eat the cottonseed until it made them sick. They tried to feed cottonseed to guinea pigs but the guinea pigs also refused to eat it.

The first of these experiments involved feeding rabbits various fractions of cottonseed which contained gossypol. The researchers literally watched the rabbits die within days.

Withers and Carruth then extracted the gossypol and other poisons from cottonseed and force fed it to four rabbits. (We can't know at this time how pure this "extract" was.) All of the rabbits died within hours. Upon autopsy, the researchers found that the dead rabbits had congested lungs. The researchers then injected this same gossypol extract to five additional rabbits. All five died within hours. Again, autopsy showed that the lungs were congested. The researchers next then fed this gossypol extract mixed in with other food. All four rabbits died with days. Autopsy showed that these animals had congested livers and lungs and also blood clots in their hearts. They fed another rabbit this same extract, instead of in a measured quantity, as much as it would eat. This rabbit died in 9 days.

Withers and Carruth then purified the "gossypol" extract further and fed it to six rabbits. All died within 35 days. Their intestines showed hemorrhage (bleeding). Lungs were congested and there were blood clots in the heart.

Next, Withers and Carruth purified the gossypol extract further, finally getting to what they thought was pure gossypol. They injected gossypol directly into the bellies of four rabbits and fed the poison to eight rabbits. The injections killed the four rabbits within hours. Of the rabbits fed this gossypol extract, six of the eight rabbits died within 55 days. The other two became ill but recovered when allowed to eat regular food. The next experiment involved feeding cottonseed to two cockerels and one chicken. They all died within days.

Withers and Carruth then went on to feed one of the residues of their purifications of cottonseed, from which they thought they had removed most of the toxic part, the "gossypol extract". Nine of 17 rabbits died within 45 days on this residue. The researchers noted that this residue also contained some gossypol and probably other poisons also. They could not get rid of all of the gossypol. More than half of the rabbits died as noted.

Based on all of these experiments, Withers and Carruth (1915) concluded that "the feeding experiments show that gossypol is very poisonous." They also could not conclude that gossypol was the only toxic compound in cottonseed. There had to be more toxic chemicals in cottonseed than gossypol.

2. *Withers and Carruth (1918): cottonseed is toxic to rats and pigs*

Withers and Carruth followed up their 1915 study with another publication in 1918.[63]

In this 1918 study, Withers and Carruth fed both raw cottonseed kernels and separately "gossypol extract" to rats. The rats died. The researchers fed the "gossypol extract" to pigs. The pigs sickened, but the researchers stopped feeding the cottonseed before the pigs actually died.

Again, Withers and Carruth concluded that gossypol is very poisonous."

3. Clark (1927): Effects of cottonseed on blood clotting

Most post 1918 researchers wanted to determine exactly how much cottonseed could be fed to animals without killing them. The researchers did not report as graphically on the specific types of problems that cottonseed toxins caused. They focused instead on growth rates of animals fed cottonseed. There are several studies that are of note however.

First, I will discuss studies on blood clotting. In Chapter 2, I discussed how cottonseed toxins interfere with blood clotting. In addition to Withers and Carruth, three additional studies show that cottonseed causes bleeding and blood clotting problems in rabbits.

Clark (1927) continued the work of Withers and Carruth. Clark, a USDA researcher, was funded in part by the Interstate Cottonseed Crushers Association. Clark studied the structure of gossypol.[64] He further purified gossypol. He injected the purified gossypol at 10 to 20 mg/kg into rats and found that they died fairly rapidly within hours to days. Autopsy findings showed that the rats had hemorrhage (bleeding) throughout their gut, heart dilatation (hearts are usually firm and muscular) and congested lungs (lungs normally have air in them rather than fluid). Clark fed animals at a lower level and a higher level. The lower level resulted in a more chronic type of poisoning. The rats exposed to chronic poisoning survived longer, but still died. The pathology at death was a little different. These chronically poisoned rats had intestinal impaction (nothing was moving). In other words, both acutely and chronically, gossypol was very toxic.

4. *Harms and Holley (1951): gossypol causes bleeding*

Harms and Holley, in 1951, also showed that cottonseed causes problems with blood clotting.[65] These investigators noted that gossypol seemed to cause hemorrhage (bleeding). They noted that rabbits fed 20% cottonseed meal in their diets developed hemorrhages not only of the intestines but also in their bones, heart muscle and around the brain. These researchers measured the clotting time in rabbits fed 20% cottonseed meal. They could not clot their blood as well as normal (the clotting time increased). The rabbits began dying around the end of the third week. They continued to die even though the clotting time started to get better around 28 days of feeding gossypol. Vitamin K (used in liver disease when there is a blood clotting problem) did not help. The animals still died. The effect of gossypol is quicker than that for dicumarol. Dicumarol is also known in various forms as coumadin and Warfarin. Warfarin is a rat poison that causes rats to die from internal bleeding.

5. *Hale and Lyman (1957): Cottonseed toxins cause heart failure and lung congestion in pigs*

Hale and Lyman published, in 1957,[66] research mainly conducted on pigs. Like Withers and Carruth, Hale and Lyman found that pigs were sensitive to gossypol or cottonseed. Hale and Lyman found that when cottonseed is fed in too great a quantity to pigs, the pigs get water in the chest, congestion and swelling (edema) of the lungs, water in the sac around the heart, swelling of the gallbladder, congestion of liver and kidney, and failing hearts. They found that the hearts were flabby and dilated. Most of the liver was not viable (Hale and Lyman, 1957). These findings extended the findings by Withers and Carruth (1918).

6. Eagle (1948): cottonseed pigment glands cause heart problems and bleeding

Eagle (1948)[67] force-fed animals the pigment glands of the cottonseed. Pigment glands are the cottonseed part in which gossypol as well as other toxins are located as well as some other toxins. The animals died. On autopsy, the researchers found that the dead animals had blood in the gut and kidneys. One of the animals had died of a heart attack (a stopped heart). Eagle and his group also found that rats were much less sensitive to the toxicity of cottonseed pigment glands than were mice, rabbits, or guinea pigs. Rats could tolerate four times as much cottonseed pigment glands as could mice. Rabbits and guinea pigs were even more sensitive.

One thing to note from this study, in addition to the findings above, is that if cottonseed meal or pigment glands are added to the diet, that diet will contain more toxins than will adding gossypol alone.

7. Boatner (1948): Cottonseed pigment glands increase toxicity and cause chicks to die

Boatner also showed in 1948[68] that adding cottonseed pigment glands to diets of chicks caused many deaths and growth retardation. An equivalent amount of gossypol (pure without all the other toxins in the pigment glands) caused many fewer problems and had little effect on growth.

This study shows that cottonseed pigment glands are much more toxic than gossypol alone because cottonseed pigment glands contain more toxins than only gossypol.

8. *Albrecht: gossypol and cottonseed meal affect heart rhythms and membrane permeability*

The next two studies show the effect of gossypol and cottonseed meal on the rhythm of the heart. From these two studies, researchers inferred that gossypol could cause changes in membrane permeability, which is also thought to be important in Alzheimer's.

Albrecht (1968)[69] fed swine cottonseed meal at about four times the level swine can tolerate. These researchers then looked at the electrocardiogram (EKG), a measure of the electrical activity of the heart. The EKG showed increased amplitude of T waves and a decrease in the ST interval. These are abnormal findings of the electrical activity of the heart. The authors noted that these changes have been observed in human beings with hyperkalemia (high potassium) and they suggested the cause to be shifts in intracellular potassium resulting from changes in membrane permeability. In clinical terms, when the potassium goes too high, people suffer from rhythm problems of the heart and die.

9. *Morgan (1988): free gossypol kills lambs; free gossypol ends up in organ meat; first researcher to recommend that people not eat cottonseed oil in combination with animal organ meat*

Morgan et al, 1988, fed free gossypol to lambs.[70] To understand why this is important, understand that in cottonseed, some gossypol is free and some is bound. Tests measuring gossypol in animal tissues showed some gossypol to be free and some to be bound. Free gossypol is much more toxic to animals than bound gossypol. Animals which have a rumen, meaning more than one stomach, such as cows, can detoxify at least partially the free gossypol because it becomes bound gossypol in the rumen (the first stomach). Lambs do not yet have this active rumen, so they cannot handle the free gossypol. Even so, at that time cottonseed was sometimes included in rations fed to lambs.

At a study site in Oklahoma in 1985, some lambs which were being fed cottonseed died. So Morgan fed free gossypol to lambs to see what would happen. She and her colleagues fed 1800 ppm (parts per million) gossypol to five lambs for 30 days. They could not complete the study, because all of the lambs were dead by the day 17. In a second experiment, Morgan decided to feed a lower amount of gossypol. They fed 20 lambs either gossypol at 100 ppm (parts per million), 300 ppm or 900 ppm or a control diet without gossypol. The goal was to feed all of the lambs for 30 days. Again, they could not complete the study on lambs fed 900 ppm gossypol. All of those lambs were dead before 30 days. The animals that died had enlarged, damaged hearts, and problems with the lungs and livers. There was fluid around the heart and around the lungs. Their lungs, trachea and bronchi were filled with red tinged froth. The EKG showed changes characteristic of increased potassium. The other animals survived for 30 days, which was the length of the study. The authors noted that others have suggested the gossypol changes the flow of fluids within cells. One of the enzymes which helps the cells produce energy was inhibited. The baby lambs died of heart failure. The authors noted that 100 ppm of gossypol was the most that could be fed to lambs, which is about the same level from other studies which can be fed to pigs. The gossypol poisoning was not immediate. The animals fed the higher level of gossypol looked fine at one week, but by one month, they were all dead.

Morgan found many of the same problems as other researchers, including heart failure. These authors recommended that lambs not receive any cottonseed until they are at least four months of age. If they receive cottonseed before that, even if they do not die, then they may have damaged hearts which may never recover. Not only did cottonseed cause heart failure, but the toxins also caused infertility. Morgan also found high concentrations of gossypol in the organs of the animals, especially the liver and kidney.

Noteworthy is that these are the first authors to extend their findings to suggestions for our diet. They recommended that people not eat a combination of cottonseed oil and organ meats, such as kidney and liver and heart, from animals known to be fed cottonseed. These organs, especially liver and kidney, contained high gossypol concentrations. Morgan also noted that gossypol causes infertility.

10. Gossypol causes male infertility

Morgan (above) observed that gossypol causes male infertility. Other researchers have noted that male rats fed cottonseed were infertile.[71] Medrano and Andreu (1986)[72] also were concerned about gossypol possibly causing male infertility. They showed that gossypol interferes with microtubules in spermatogenesis, the formation of sperm. These investigators found that gossypol binds to microtubules in the male system and inhibits microtubule assembly as sperm are being formed. In other words, gossypol prevents the formation of sperm. This interferes with fertility. The Chinese experimented with gossypol as a way of temporary birth control for men. However, gossypol caused permanent infertility in some men.[73]

11. Gossypol binds to proteins in such a way as to cause neurofibrillary tangles, a major lesion of Alzheimer's disease

Other researchers have also found that gossypol has been shown binds to proteins in such a way that might cause neurofibrillary tangles, one of the major lesions of Alzheimer's. When scientists have studied the neurofibrillary tangles from Alzheimer's patients, they have found cross links between proteins at sites of glutamine and lysine residues (glutamine and lysine are parts of protein).[74] When looking at gossypol, researchers have found that gossypol contains a number of free carbonyl groups and phenolic groups (reactive chemical groups).[75] These reactive groups bind to a number of amino acids, especially the epsilon-amino groups of lysine residues (a particular binding site on an important amino acid or part of protein).[76] In other words, gossypol binds to proteins in all the right places where neurofibrillary tangles are bound[77]. Cater and Lyman (1969)[78] showed that gossypol also complexes with other amino acid residues, including glutamine residues. In addition, Lyman, Baliga and Slay (1959)[79] showed that gossypol has been shown to cross link proteins, resulting in decreased enzymatic activity (the protein was not working).

The effect of these studies is to show that gossypol deactivates proteins by binding to them. Deactivation of proteins was important in researching animal feed because deactivated protein has less nutritional value than normal protein. However, gossypol also binds to proteins in the same places as we find for binding in the neurofibrillary tangles of Alzheimer's.

The studies on protein deactivation and neurofibrillary tangles have important implications for Alzheimer's. Gossypol could well be involved in binding to the proteins in such a way that causes neurofibrillary tangles, a major lesion and sign of Alzheimer's.

12. Accumulation of gossypol

By the early 1960's, scientists developed measurement techniques to study how much gossypol was present in the muscle and other tissues of animals fed cottonseed.[80] The first such report was in pigs. The amount of gossypol found in muscle was about 4 to 8 ppm (parts per million). The muscle has some of the smallest amounts of all of the organs tested. The liver contained 100 times the amount found in muscle. Kidneys also had large amounts. This study also showed that gossypol was reaching the brain. Even pigs' brains had a little more than muscle at about 8 ppm.[81]

13. Genotoxic effects

Gossypol is known to damage DNA. Gossypol causes DNA strand breaks and exchange of genetic material across chromosomes.[82] Both of these effects can result in significant genetic mutations. The integrity of DNA is exceedingly important to human beings. We need our DNA to stay intact throughout life. Yet, in our food, we are taking in a "genotoxic" chemical. We have little idea exactly how significant gossypol's damage to DNA may be. However, we do know there are disorders such as autism, which are more likely when the father is older. Such effects are thought to be due to the accumulation of "spontaneous" genetic mutations as the father ages.[83] But these mutations may not be spontaneous. They may be induced by gossypol intake and accumulation throughout life.

The effects of gossypol on DNA may be one of the worst things gossypol does because such effects cause major problems in the next generation. We won't know for sure until more research is done.

Toxicity of cyclopropenoid fatty acids

In addition to gossypol, cottonseeds contain another pair of poisons which are very significant, called the cyclopropenoid fatty acids (CPFA's). One can find these acids primarily in the oil after the cottonseed is pressed to separate oil from the cottonseed meal.

Thus, every time a person consumes cottonseed oil, that person is consuming CPFA's directly.

1. Discoloration in eggs: because cottonseed causes discoloration of eggs, egg-laying chickens are not fed cottonseed

Research on CPFA's goes back to the 1930's and to the concern about pink eggs. When hens are fed cottonseed meal, the eggs develop a pink color, which is not aesthetically pleasing. Worse yet, the eggs also can also develop a brown olive color. The cause of this pink color problem was found to be due to the CPFA's.[84] The brown olive color was found to be due to gossypol in the cottonseed meal. Researchers identified these two types of discoloration as "pink white" problems and browning in eggs. The problem of how to avoid this discoloration was one that cottonseed researchers never solved, except by avoiding cottonseed. The end result was that cottonseed could not be fed to chickens which lay eggs.

2. Cottonseed oil and CPFA's raise cholesterol even though it contains polyunsaturated fatty acids

In the late 1950's researchers had found that cholesterol may be important in heart disease. They further found that some polyunsaturated fatty acids lower cholesterol. Because cottonseed oil contains large amounts of polyunsaturated fatty acids, researchers studied whether cottonseed oil would help lower cholesterol. To the dismay of cottonseed researchers, cottonseed oil has the opposite effect. Instead of lowering cholesterol, cottonseed oil actually raises cholesterol.

Tennent et al. (1959)[85] found that cottonseed oil uniformly produced high blood plasma cholesterol concentrations in cockerels (a type of poultry) fed cottonseed oil. This finding was surprising at the time because cottonseed oil contains high levels of polyunsaturated fatty acids. Other vegetable oils which contain high levels of polyunsaturated fatty acids lower cholesterol. Tennent found that hens fed cottonseed oil had higher serum cholesterol levels and a greater degree of atherosclerosis than would have been predicted from the content of saturated fatty acids in the oil.[86] These researchers hypothesized that something else in cottonseed oil raises plasma cholesterol.

By 1960, researchers found that cottonseed oil contains CPFA's.[87] These acids were found to be responsible for causing "pink white" disorder in eggs. Did they also increase plasma cholesterol?

Goodknight and Kemmerer (1967)[88] tested the hypothesis that the CPFA's in cottonseed oil increases plasma cholesterol. They fed either cottonseed oil or CPFA's to cockerels and found that CPFA's, either pure, or as part of cottonseed oil, both increased plasma cholesterol concentrations and caused atherosclerosis in cockerels. These researchers concluded that CPFA was the chemical in cottonseed oil which increased cholesterol.

Researchers found the same effect in mammals. Ferguson, et. al., (1976)[89] found that CPFA caused atherosclerotic heart disease and increased cholesterol in rabbits. Matlock and Nixon (1986)[90] showed that CPFA in concentrated quantities caused increased cholesterol in mice.

3. CPFA's work to cause increased cholesterol by interfering with the body's ability to excrete cholesterol

To understand why CPFA's cause increased cholesterol, even though cottonseed oil contains polyunsaturated fatty acids, one needs to understand something about how the body handles and excretes cholesterol. Excretion of cholesterol requires several steps. First, the body needs to bind cholesterol to certain structures before it can be excreted. The body cannot clear pure cholesterol as pure cholesterol. The structures to which the body binds cholesterol also contain unsaturated fatty acids. This process of binding the cholesterol converts cholesterol, a saturated fat, into a less saturated fat. If the cells cannot do this, then cholesterol cannot be excreted as easily. If the body's cells do not have enough unsaturated fatty acids, then the cholesterol will not be bound at all or will be bound up with saturated fatty acids and will be harder to excrete.

Research shows that the CPFA's in cottonseed inhibit the body from desaturating (converting saturated fatty acids to unsaturated fatty acids) fatty acids. Reiser and Raju, 1964,[91] and Johnson, et. al., 1967[92] found that CPFA inhibit fatty acid desaturation by inhibiting the stearoyl-CoA-delta9-monodesaturase enzyme (an enzyme which converts a saturated fat to an unsaturated fat), which in turn leads to an imbalance of saturated fat to unsaturated fat. Then unsaturated fatty acids are not available to bind for cholesterol excretion which in turn leads to an imbalance of cholesterol esters. Then cholesterol increases because it is bound to the wrong fatty acids and cannot be excreted.

In summary, the cottonseed poisons CPFA inhibit the body from desaturating fatty acids, so then unsaturated fatty acids are not available to bind for cholesterol excretion and cholesterol increases.

Matlock and Nixon (1986)[93] researched the question of whether the effect of CPFA's on enzymes translates into higher cholesterol and lesions of atherosclerosis in the arteries. Matlock and Nixon fed mice CPFA's as 0.7% of their diets for eight weeks. They found an increase in the proportion of saturated fat which was bound to cholesterol and a decrease in the amount of cholesterol which was excreted, when a labeled cholesterol load was given. This shows that when mice are fed CPFA's, they do not excrete all of their cholesterol.

Ferguson (1976)[94] fed CPFA to rabbits at 0.27% of the diet with or without added cholesterol of the diet for five weeks. By week 3, the cholesterol in rabbits fed the CPFA had doubled and by week 5, the cholesterol of the CPFA fed rabbits was three times as high as rabbits fed the control diet. Plasma triglycerides were also higher in the rabbits fed CPFA. Liver cholesterol also increased and the percentage of free cholesterol as opposed to bound cholesterol increased. These researchers also looked for plaques in the arteries. Five of the eight rabbits fed CPFA had early lesions of atherosclerosis in only five weeks. Rabbits fed cholesterol plus CPFA had much more extensive atherosclerosis in their aortas in only five weeks. These researchers also found that CPFA accumulated in the fat on the animals to 2% in only five weeks.

In summary, the research shows that CPFA interfere with excretion of cholesterol and in a very short period of time can cause atherosclerosis in rabbits.

4. CPFA's cause cancer and collects in the animals' organs

CPFA's caused liver cancer in rainbow trout (Ayres, et al, 1971).[95] Eisele and coworker (1982)[96] fed CPFA to rabbits as part of a cancer study. The rabbits did not gain as much weight as they should have. Their growth was slowed. As part of this study, the investigators measured the amount of CPFA's in the tissues. CPFA's were found in all organs in the fat. In 28 days in rabbits, the adipose fat tissue contained 14.7% CPFA's. Kidney fat contained 1.1% and liver fat contained 2.8%. These studies show that CPFA accumulates in the fat in animals which receive CPFA in the diet. These numbers are enormous amounts of CPFA in the fat, showing that CPFA remains in the animal fat. 14.7% CPFA means that CPFA has shifted the composition of the animal fat.

Other studies have shown that CPFA is present in animal fat. A study in 1971 shows CPFA's in the fat of fish.[97] The researchers fed CPFA at 0, 100 ppm, or 200 ppm, to rainbow trout and found that the amount of CPFA approached 0.1% to 0.2% of the total lipid (fat).[98] This is a higher percentage than found in the dairy fat, and shows that the fish do not clear the CPFAs. The amounts found in the rabbits are higher numbers than in the fish.

In another study, Hawkins et. al., (1985) measured CPFA in milk from dairy cows fed cottonseed. These researchers found CPFA quantity of 59.6 mg/g dairy fat.[99]

So in this study the dairy fat portion of the diet is 0.006% CPFA. In fish fat, the percentage may be 0.1% and in unrefined cottonseed oil, the percentage is 1.5%. The rabbit study showing 14.7% in the fat of rabbits shows that the percentages can go even higher.

In other words, the amounts of CPFA found in animal fats and other tissues could be quite high, which could result in high intakes of CPFA in human beings.

The biggest issues with CPFA research was that it came to an abrupt halt. Despite the possibility of showing that CPFA may be contributing to human coronary artery disease, the research came to an end. I talked with one researcher in about 1990, a few years after this research stopped. He was a toxicologist and said his grants were not renewed. He went to work as a toxicologist for a large company.

In an earlier chapter, we reviewed how much CPFA is in the diet versus how much caused heart disease in the rats in the experiment described here. As noted in chapter 5, there is plenty of CPFA in the human diet to be causing heart disease.

APPENDIX B

RESEARCHING COTTONSEED: A SUGGESTION FOR A MORE COLLABORATIVE APPROACH

Issues of diet and health would be much better studied if our biomedical research community worked in a more cooperative way. However, diet is not on the radar screen for most doctors and for the biomedical research community. Should it be? Are there really enough poisons out there to be worth studying, either at all or as the potential cause of diseases? The answer is yes, as indicated by the findings above on cottonseed. There are dietary poisons in our food which are worth studying. But the research community is not studying dietary poisons. There are no University departments devoted to these subjects. Diet is not important in the medical community. There are toxic chemicals in foods but there is no place which even collects a total list of all such chemicals, let alone makes any attempt to determine the impact of all these chemicals.

In addition, we have a very competitive scientific system. Scientists are competing for limited funds. As noted in an earlier chapter, while in theory this should produce the best ideas, such as system also leads to lack of risk taking because no one wants to be on the outside trying to get back in.

What if science was more cooperative? What if groups of scientists came together and tried to find answers collectively.

Let us start looking for answers as to why dietary poisons are not being studied.

Today, researchers in different labs compete to be the first in new findings and especially in the seeking of research money. Again, as noted in an earlier chapter, while this may work for narrow questions, large questions would be difficult to research in a competitive way because more than a single laboratory would have to be involved.

Let us imagine that researchers worked in a cooperative way and did not worry about who receives credit for findings. Instead, they would work to find answers to questions. Let us imagine a meeting based on cooperation.

What if a meeting were held to look for the cause of Alzheimer's?

One way to look for possible causes of Alzheimer's disorder would be to hold a meeting of a diverse group of scientists. People who study the lesions of Alzheimer's would be invited but also scientists who study other problems as well as other health care practitioners and members of the public. Then this group would brainstorm and try to come up with as many possible Alzheimer's causes as possible. All the ideas would be written on a blackboard. So someone might suggest that the cause is pesticide and insecticide residues and someone else might say vitamin deficiencies. Another might say toxic chemicals from air pollution. Another might say, old age or lack of exercise. The Alzheimer's researchers would say that they are identifying important genes so perhaps some kind of defective genes are the cause. Then some public member might say that the brain needs stem cells as it grows older. Another person might suggest toxic metals such as mercury, lead or aluminum.

Someone else might say that the cause is toxic chemicals in food and someone might say well what would they be? Perhaps it's all those food additives and food colorings.

I learned in an engineering class that one should not exclude anything on such initial lists. So let us look at the list so far.

A list of possible Alzheimer's causes could be developed

✓ Pesticide and insecticide residues

✓ vitamin deficiencies, mineral deficiencies, other nutritional deficiencies

✓ lack of exercise,

✓ simple old age,

✓ toxic chemicals from air pollution,

✓ food colorings and food additives,

✓ Toxic chemicals from food.

✓ Toxic metals such as mercury, lead or aluminum

✓ Intellectual stagnation, brain cells simply degenerate spontaneously

✓ Defective genes, lack of the right drugs for the brain

✓ Lack of stem cells as we become older

✓ Alcohol, drug abuse, other prescription drugs,

✓ Lack of oxygen or some other waste chemical from organ malfunction in the body, such as kidneys or liver.

✓ I'm sure that you can think of other possible causes but let me suggest another set of possibilities.

What about possible toxic chemicals in food?

What if someone asked do we really know everything toxic that is contained within food? The answer to this would have to be no, as very few people study toxic chemicals in food. There is no government agency concerned with toxic chemicals in food that appear naturally and there are no University departments of the diet. So now we can add to the list chemical carcinogens, bacterial poisons from food poisoning such as Salmonella and fungal poisons. There are chemicals in foods such as vinegar, chocolate, cheese and malt.

And then there's one more group of chemicals which would be brought out only if a veterinarian was in the group. If someone were to ask are there any toxic chemicals which are fed to animals, which human beings then consume. What about all the hormone residues in meat and antibiotics fed to animals? These might be a possibility. Are there other toxic chemicals which are fed to farm animals? Then the veterinarian might say that cottonseed is fed very heavily to animals. "Does it contain anything toxic?" someone asks. "Well yes it does", replies the veterinarian. "It contains gossypol, a toxic chemical that affects blood clotting." "Does it reach the brain?" "Yes it does." "Does it bind in the brain?" "Yes, it does." "Can the body get rid of it?" "The body cannot clear it very well." "Does it tie things together?" "Yes it does." "Is it there in large quantities?" "Relatively for a poison, it is quite present."

The idea that chemicals may be present in animal feed, which remain in the meat and fat of the animal and are then consumed by human beings, opens up many possibilities. Would such chemicals be known to the biomedical research community? No. Biomedical researchers are concerned about medical problems. Agricultural researchers look at such chemicals because they are part of the problem of feeding animals. If you feed something toxic to an animal, that animal won't grow and that is an agricultural problem.

Now we have a possibility, something besides defective genes. We have a poison in our food, which reaches the brain, binds randomly, that we cannot get rid of and is present in fairly large quantities in food.

Other toxic chemicals might play some role but the cottonseed poison gossypol on first glance looks like a possibility that should be tested.

The possible further value of such a meeting

If we now extend the value of such a meeting, the next step would be to determine which ideas have been tested and which ideas are worth testing further. People familiar with looking through scientific studies would then have to go through everything known about what causes Alzheimer's, which possibilities have been investigated and ruled out and which ones should be tested further.

If this step were to be taken, the answer would be that toxic chemicals in food have not been researched thoroughly. Why? Gathering such information is hard. Studies of toxic chemicals to be worthwhile would have to use levels that human beings are actually exposed to, something which is almost never done. Given that there are few studies to go on, the group would have to decide what is worth looking at further.

The next step would be for the group to give out money so that important possibilities could be investigated.

Such an approach seems reasonable and should help in the finding of the cause of Alzheimer's. Would such a meeting ever take place?

Such a meeting has not occurred

Such a meeting has never been held and never would be held under the current way scientists organize themselves. There is no one at the top directing larger numbers of scientists, looking for all the possibilities, then trying to find the best one, or to find ideas worth testing. No such collaborative meetings are held. As noted in an earlier chapter, each scientist tries to come up with a project that other scientists think have some merit. While this in theory should produce good ideas also, such a system is very unlikely to come up with a research idea which requires much collaboration across disciplines.

But we noted in Chapter 8 that researching a dietary cause of Alzheimer's requires much collaboration across disciplines.

The illustration of this collaborative meeting shows that many different ideas would be produced in such a meeting. The idea that maybe cottonseed toxins such as gossypol play a role in causing Alzheimer's might come out in such a meeting. But in the single discipline lab system such an idea is unlikely to come out. The amount of collaboration and knowledge about other disciplines required would make it unlikely that this idea would come out.

There should be such collaborative meetings.

APPENDIX C

CANCER CAUSING FOODS YOU SHOULD AVOID

Although this book is mainly about the effects of cottonseed poisons, I wish to give some information about cancer causers in the diet. After I completed medical school and internship, I studied for a PhD at the University of California-Davis. I studied protein nutrition. Then I went to work at a laboratory at the National Cancer Institute concerned with diet and cancer prevention. There I studied various chemicals in food which cause cancer. I became interested in the cottonseed poisons because they were on some of the lists of foods which affect the genes or cause cancer. One of the major cancer causers, benzo(a)pyrene (discussed below) and gossypol are about the same size and both go everywhere in the body. Let us look at cancer causers in the diet.

I ask this hypothetical question. You are 30 years old and you recently found out that your mother at age 57 has been diagnosed with breast cancer. Do you change anything about your eating because of your mother's diagnosis? I think that if you called the National Cancer Institute and asked, no one could give you a complete, easy to follow or understand answer.

But there is an answer. When I was at the National Cancer Institute in 1989, I looked at cancer causing chemicals in foods. The first chemicals I looked at were the polycyclic aromatic hydrocarbons. These are chemicals which form when there is incomplete combustion or burning. When there is smoke, there is incomplete burning. The best known examples of such chemicals are the chemicals in cigarette smoke, commonly referred to as tar. These are polycyclic aromatic hydrocarbons, of which benzo(a)pyrene is one. These chemicals are very potent at causing cancer. They look like cholesterol, so the body pumps them everywhere. They also last in the body a long time and they taste good.

The other main place (besides cigarettes) people take in such chemicals is from food cooked over charcoal grills and also from gas grills. Whenever meat fat spatters over the grill and causes smoke, these chemicals are formed. I read everything I could find about such chemicals. In addition, I read reports about all the chemicals people thought might be important in human cancer. I concluded that the polycyclic aromatic hydrocarbons had to be important because none of the other chemicals mentioned as causing cancer were as potent and long lasting as the polycyclic aromatic hydrocarbons. For example some of the other chemicals which cause cancer only last a minute in the body. Polycyclic aromatic hydrocarbons can last a month. These chemicals are present in our diets because they taste good.

Let us look at why these chemicals should be feared especially if you have a family history of cancer. One fact which is not widely known but is publicly available is how much cancer causer there is in a piece of meat which has been charcoal grilled. The charcoal grilling of a 1.1 kg, (a little over 2 pounds) steak leads to the production of a number of cancer causing polycyclic aromatic hydrocarbons including the representative chemical benzo(a)pyrene. There is enough cancer causing chemical in this 1.1 kg steak to be equal to the cancer causing chemical amount in 600 cigarettes.[100] This means that eating this steak once a month means that a person is taking in the equivalent amount of cancer causer as someone smoking 1 pack of cigarettes per day. And this person only needs to do this once per month. Twice a month would be equivalent to two packs of cigarettes per day. Remember that the body pumps these chemicals everywhere, so they could cause any type of cancer.

Should we wonder why we have a cancer problem in this country? There are many people who eat this kind of meat regularly. And they are regularly taking in large quantities of cancer causing chemicals.

So what is the answer to the question of what the 30 year old should do and what all of us who are concerned about cancer should do. The answer is that the 30 year old should not smoke, not eat charcoal grilled or gas grilled meat, and should not eat smoked foods. Smoked foods also contain large quantities of these chemicals.[101]

I think that there would be far less cancer in this country if these simple rules were followed.

No amount of supplements or other dietary changes have ever been shown to protect against such chemicals.

APPENDIX D

THE HIGH MEDICAL COSTS OF COTTONSEED IN OUR DIET

As noted in earlier chapters, the use of cottonseed as animal feed results in cottonseed toxins entering the animals. Humans then eat these cottonseed toxins throughout life which results in major medical problems such as Alzheimer's, bleeding and heart disease. Even though cottonseed feeding results in major health problems, the government of the United States subsidizes the production of cotton to an amount of between $1 billion and $3 billion per year.[102] This subsidy results in more cotton being grown and more cottonseed is then available for animal feed. This means that the cotton subsidy results in more cottonseed toxins entering human beings every year than there would be if there was no subsidy. These extra cottonseed toxins result in more health problems than there would be without a cotton subsidy.

How much extra health care cost might the use of cottonseed in agriculture be causing? The cost of Alzheimer's care is $200 billion per year.[103] The cost of heart disease care is $444 billion.[104] We don't know with certainty how much cottonseed is contributing to these disorders. If the amount were only 25% of $200 billion and $444 billion, this would be $161 billion in disease care costs. This number may be too low as an estimate because cottonseed toxins may be the major cause of both Alzheimer's and high cholesterol and atherosclerotic heart disease. But even at 25% and $161 billion in disease care costs, how do these numbers compare with the total value of the cottonseed crop in the United States.

The total cottonseed production in the United States is 5 to 6 million tons per year. The cost of a ton of cottonseed is around $300.[105] The cost of the entire cottonseed crop is on the order of $1.8 billion. Conservatively, this number is 1.1% of the disease care costs of $161 billion. In other words, the loss to the government and to the economy and insurance companies is at least 90 times higher in health care costs than the entire value of the cottonseed crop.

These numbers mean that if the government bought the entire cottonseed crop and turned it into diesel fuel, the government would benefit in lower health care costs by 90 fold, and perhaps much more. Nothing that the government does yields a 90 fold return or higher as easily as prohibiting the use of cottonseed in agriculture. Cottonseed better belongs in the diesel fuel tank, not in our food.

INDEX

FOOTNOTES AND ENDNOTES

Chapter 1:

1   Semon, B. A. Dietary Intake of Cottonseed Toxins is hypothesized to be a partial cause of Alzheimer's disorder. Medical Hypotheses. Feb. 2012. V.78(2):293-298.

2   http://www.cotton.com

3   http://www.cottonseed.com/publications/feedproducts-guide.asp; 1/2/12

4   Withers, W. A., and Carruth, F. E., (1915) Gossypol, The toxic substance in cottonseed meal. J. Agric. Research, 5(7): 261-283.

Chapter 2:

5   Withers, W. A., and Carruth, F. E., (1915) Gossypol, The toxic substance in cottonseed meal. J. Agric. Research,; 5(7): 261-283.

6   Clark, E. P., (1927) Studies on Gossypol. I. The preparation, purification, and some of the properties of gossypol, the toxic principle of cottonseed. J. Biol Chem. 75:725-739.

7   Eagle, E., Castillon, L. E., Hall, C. M., and C. H. Boatner. (1948) Acute Oral Toxicity of Gossypol and Cottonseed pigment Glands for Rats, Mice, Rabbits, and Guinea Pigs. Arch. Biochem. 18: 271-277.

8   Harms, W. S., and K. T. Holley. (1951) Hypoprothrombinemia Induced by Gossypol. Proc. Soc. For Experimental Biology and Medicine.; 77:297-299.

9 Tennent, D. M., Zanetti, M. E., Siegel, H., Kuron, G. W and Ott, W. H. (1959). The influence of selected vegetable fats on plasma lipid concentrations and aortic atheromatosis in cholesterol-fed and diethylstilbestrol-implanted cockerels. J. Nutrition. 69, 283-88.

10 Reiser, R., and Raju, P. K. (1964). The inhibition of saturated fatty acid dehydrogenation by dietary fat containing sterculic and malvalic acids. Biochem. Biophys. Res. Commun. 17:8-11.

Johnson, A. R., Person, J. A. Shenstone, F. S. and Fogerty, A. C. (1967). Inhibition of the desaturation of stearic to oleic acid by cylopropene fatty acid. Nature (London) 214:1244-1245.

11 Ferguson, T.L., Wales, J.H., Sinnhuber, R. O. and D. J. Lee. (1976) Cholesterol Levels, Atherosclerosis and Liver morphology in rabbits fed cyclopropenoid fatty acids. Food Cosmetology and Toxicology. 14:15-18.

12 Matlock, J. P., and J. E. Nixon. (1986). Impaired Clearance, Elimination, and Metabolism of Plasma Cholesterol Esters Associated with Hypercholesteremia in Mice Fed Cyclopropenoid Fatty Acids. Toxicology and Applied Pharmacology. 84:3-11.

13 http://www.framinghamheartstudy.org/about/milestones. html, http://www.nhlbi.nih.gov/about/framingham/index.hm

14 Hu, F. B., Stampfer, M. J., Rimm, E. B, Manson, J. E., Ascherio, A., Colditz, G. A., Rosner, B. A., Spiegelman, D., Speizer, F. E., Sacks, F. M., Ehnnekens, C. H., and W. C. Willett. (1999) A Prospective Study of Egg Consumption and Risk of Cardiovascular Disease in Men and Women. JAMA; 281(15): 1387-1394.

15 Phelps, R. A., Shenstone, F. S. Kemmerer, AR, Evans, R.J. (1964) A review of cyclopropenoid compounds: biological effect of some derivatives. Poult Sci. 44:358-94.

16 Ambrose, A. M., and D. J. Robbins. (1951) Studies on the chronic oral toxicity of cottonseed meal and cottonseed pigment glands. J. Nutrition. 43:357-70.

17 Medrano, F. J., Andreu, J.M. (1986) Binding of gossypol to purified tubulin and inhibition of its assembly into microtubules. Eur. J. Biochem. 1986; 158(1):63-9

18 Ibid.

19 Eagle, E., Castillon, L. E., Hall, C. M., and C. H. Boatner. (1948) Acute Oral Toxicity of Gossypol and Cottonseed pigment Glands for Rats, Mice, Rabbits, and Guinea Pigs. Arch. Biochem. 18: 271-277.

20 Boatner, C. H., In: Bailey, A. E., editor. Cottonseed and cottonseed products: their chemistry and chemical technology. New York: Wiley (Interscience); 1948, p 213-362 (Chapter 6).

Chapter 3:

21 Smith, F.H., and A. J. Clawson. (1965) Effect of Diet on Accumulation of Gossypol in the Organs of Swine. Journal of Nutrition. 87: 317-321.

22 De la Torre, J.C. (2006) How do heart disease and stroke become risk factors for Alzheimer's disease. Neurol. Res. 28:637-644.

23 Cordonnier, C., and van der Flier, W. M. (2011) Brain Microbleeds and Alzheimer's disease: innocent observation or key player. Brain. 134:335-44.

24 Bowman, G. L. Kaye, J. A., Moore, M. Waichunas, D., Carlson, NE, Quinn, J. F. (2007) Blood-Brain barrier impairment in Alzheimer Disease: stability and functional significance. Neurology. 68:1809-1814.

25 Epidemiologically from the Adventist Health Study, reduced intake of animal products has been associated with lower risk of Alzheimer's (Giem, P. Beeson, W.L., Fraser, G. E. The incidence of dementia and intake of animal products: preliminary findings from the Adventist Health Study. Neuroepidemiology. 1993; 12(1):28-36). In another population control study of Alzheimer's patients, the presence of the disorder was associated with higher meat intake. Gustaw-Rothenberg, K. Dietary patterns associated with Alzheimer's disease: population based study Int J Environ Res Public Health. 2009 Apr;6(4):1335-40. Epub 2009 Apr 1. These findings are consistent with an environmental toxin found in meat products such as cottonseed toxins being ingested throughout life.

26 Medrano, F. J. and J. M. Andreu. (1986) Binding of gossypol to purified tubulin and inhibition of its assembly into microtubules. Eur. J. Biochem. 158(1):63-9.

27 Smith, F.H., and A. J. Clawson. Effect of Diet on Accumulation of Gossypol in the Organs of Swine. Journal of Nutrition. 87: 317-321, 1965.

Sharma, M. P., Smith, F. H. and A. J. Clawson. (1966) Effects of Levels of Protein and Gossypol, and Length of Feeding Period on the Accumulation of Gossypol in Tissues of Swine. Journal of Nutrition, 88:434-438. Other studies are discussed in the appendix.

Chapter 4:

28 Gamboa, D. A., M. C. Calhoun, Kuhlmann, S.W., Haq, A. U. and C. A. Bailey. (2001). Use of Expander Cottonseed Meal in Broiler Diets Formulated on a Digestible Amino Acid Basis. Poultry Science. 80:789-794.

Chapter 5:

29 Smith, F.H., and A. J. Clawson. (1965) Effect of Diet on Accumulation of Gossypol in the Organs of Swine. Journal of Nutrition. 87: 317-321.

30 Sharma, M. P., Smith, F. H. and A. J. Clawson. (1966) Effects of Levels of Protein and Gossypol, and Length of Feeding Period on the Accumulation of Gossypol in Tissues of Swine. Journal of Nutrition, 88:434-438.

31 Gamboa, D. A., M. C. Calhoun, Kuhlmann, S.W., Haq, A. U. and C. A. Bailey. (2001). Use of Expander Cottonseed Meal in Broiler Diets Formulated on a Digestible Amino Acid Basis. Poultry Science. 80:789-794.

32 Bouchard, M, Gosselin, N. H. R. C. Brunet, Samuel, O, Dumoilin, M-J and G. Carrier. A toxicokinetic Model of Malathion and Its Metabolites as a Tool to Assess Human Exposure and Risk through Measurement of Urinary Biomarkers. Toxicological Sciences. 73:182-194, 2003.

33 Velasquez-Pereira, J., McDowell, L. R., Risco, C.A., Prichard, D., Martin, F. G., Calhoun, M. C., Williams, S. N., Wilkinson, N. S., and P. Ogebe. (1988). Effects on Performance, Tissue Integrity, and Metabolism of Vitamin E Supplementation for Beef Heifers Fed a Diet that contains Gossypol. J. Anim. Sci. 76:2871-2884.

34 Roehm, J. N., Lee, D. J. and R. O. Sinnhuber. (1967). Accumulation and Elimination of Dietary Gossypol in the Organs of Rainbow Trout. Journal of Nutrition. 92: 425-428.

35 Abou-Donia, M. B. and J. W. Dieckert. (1970) Metabolic fate of gossypol: The metabolism of 14Cgossypol in rats. Lipids. 5, 938-46.

36 Sharma, M. P., Smith, F. H. and A. J. Clawson. (1966) Effects of Levels of Protein and Gossypol, and Length of Feeding Period on the Accumulation of Gossypol in Tissues of Swine. Journal of Nutrition, 1966; 88:434-438.

37 Eisele, T. A., Loveland, P. M., Kruk, D. L., Meyers, T. R., Sinnhuber, R. O. and J. E. Nixon. (1982) Effect of cyclopropenoid fatty acids on the hepatic microsomal mixed-function-oxidase system and aflatoxin metabolism in rabbits. Food and Chemical Toxicology. 20:407-412. And Roehm, J. N., Lee, D. J. and R. O. Sinnhuber, and S. D. Polityka. (1971). Deposition of Cyclopropenoids in the Tissue Lipids of Rainbow Trout Fed Methyl Sterculate. Lipids. 6(6): 426-430.

38 Shenstone, F. S. and J. R. Vickery. (1961) Occurrence of Cyclo-Propene Acids in Some plants of the Order Malvales. Nature. 190:168-169.

39 The ingredients of a Dunkin' Donuts French Cruller are: Donut Dough {Water, Dough Mix {Wheat Starch, Palm Oil, Egg Yolk with Sodium Silicoaluminate, Egg Whites, Sodium Caseinate, Corn Starch, Mono and Diglycerides, Leavening (Baking Soda, Sodium Aluminum Phosphate), Salt, Whey, Soy Flour]}, Shortening (Palm Oil, Partially Hydrogenated Soybean Oil and Partially Hydrogenated Cottonseed Oil with TBHQ and Citric Acid added to help protect flavor), Glaze [Sugar, Water, Maltodextrin, Contains 2% or less of: Propylene Glycol, Mono and Diglycerides (Emulsifier), Potassium Sorbate (Preservative), Agar, Citric Acid, Carboxymethyl Cellulose, Artificial Flavor]. http://www.dunkindonuts.com/content/dunkindonuts/en/menu/donuts.html?DRP_FLAVOR=French%20Cruller, accessed 7/10/12. I am confining

my discussion here to cottonseed oil. However, note that Maltodextrin is also an ingredient in the doughnut, which is problematic for many other reasons. See Bruce Semon, M.D. and Lori Kornblum, *An Extraordinary Power to Heal* (2003) or our website, www.nutritioninstitute.com. Dunkin' Donuts and other donut manufacturers have been eliminating trans-fats from their donuts. Due to the necessity of using a fat that is solid at room temperature, Dunkin Donuts has come up with a proprietary blend that includes some cottonseed oil. They do not reveal how much cottonseed oil they use. For more information, see the following websites, accessed on 7/10/12: "The long, secret journey to a healthier donut," By Jenn Abelson, Boston Globe, September 16, 2007, http://www.boston. com/business/globe/articles/2007/09/16/the_long_secret_journey_to_a_healthier_donut/?page=full; See also information about changing the fats used to fry donuts, in "The Zero Trans-Fat Cooking Contest," Frytest.com, http://www.frytest.com/frying_donuts. php, accessed 7/10/12

40 According to the National Cottonseed Products Association, "Cottonseed oil has been a part of the American diet for well over a century. Until the 1940's, it was the major vegetable oil produced in the United States. Now, with annual production averaging more than 1 billion pounds, Cottonseed oil ranks third in volume behind soybean and corn oil representing about 5-6% of the total domestic fat and oil supply." http://www.cottonseed.com/publications/facts. asp, accessed 7/10/12.

41 "Utz" brand of potato chips has several varieties fried in pure cottonseed oil. http://www.utzsnacks.com/nutritioninfo_transfat. html, accessed 7/10/12. For the brand "Moon Brand Original Saratoga Chips," www.cottonseedoiltour.com/pdf/chip.pdf

Accessed 7/10/12. Other brands may use a blend of oils including cottonseed.

42 http://www.cottonseed.com/publications/facts.asp, accessed July 10, 2012

43 Hawkins, G.E., Cummins, K. A., Silverio, M. and J. J. Jilek. (1985). Physiological Effects of Whole Cottonseed in the Diet of Lactating Dairy Cows. J. Dairy Science. 68:2608-2614.

44 Roehm, J. N., Lee, D. J. and R. O. Sinnhuber, and S. D. Polityka. (1971). Deposition of Cyclopropenoids in the Tissue Lipids of Rainbow Trout Fed Methyl Sterculate. Lipids. 6(6): 426-430.

45 Eisele, T. A., Loveland, P. M., Kruk, D. L., Meyers, T. R., Sinnhuber, R. O. and J. E. Nixon. (1982) Effect of cyclopropenoid fatty acids on the hepatic microsomal mixed-function-oxidase system and aflatoxin metabolism in rabbits. Food and Chemical Toxicology. 20:407-412. The cyclopropenoid fatty acids used in this study come from Sterculia foetida oil which is 50% CPFA.

46 This is a nutritional calculation that is commonly used to describe the normal diet, but it excludes water.

47 The diet of a person eating one doughnut, two ¼ pound hamburgers and 1/3 stick of butter works out to be about 93 grams of fat per day or 837 calories. In a 2700 calorie diet of a hypothetical male, this would be 26.7% calories as fat. (This amount is lower than average for many people.)

Chapter 6:

48 Santos, J. E. P., Villasenor, M., Robinson, P. H., DePeters, E. J. and C. A. Holmberg. (2003). Type of Cottonseed and Level of Gossypol in Diets of Lactating Dairy Cows: Plasma Gossypol, Health, and Reproductive Performance. Journal of Dairy Science. 86:892-905.

Velasquez-Pereira, J., McDowell, L. R., Risco, C.A., Prichard, D., Martin, F. G., Calhoun, M. C., Williams, S. N., Wilkinson, N.

S., and P. Ogebe. (1988). Effects on Performance, Tissue Integrity, and Metabolism of Vitamin E Supplementation for Beef Heifers Fed a Diet that contains Gossypol. J. Anim. Sci. 76:2871-2884.

Chapter 7:

49 Withers, W. A., and Carruth, F. E., Gossypol, The toxic substance in cottonseed meal. J. Agric. Research, 1915; 5(7): 261-283; Clark, E. P. Studies on Gossypol. I. The preparation, purification, and some of the properties of gossypol, the toxic principle of cottonseed. J. Biol Chem. 1927; 75:725-739; Harms, W. S., and K. T. Holley. Hypoprothrombinemia Induced by Gossypol. Proc. Soc. For Experimental Biology and Medicine. 1951; 77:297-299; Eagle, E., Castillon, L. E., Hall, C. M., and C. H. Boatner. Acute Oral Toxicity of Gossypol and Cottonseed pigment Glands for Rats, Mice, Rabbits, and Guinea Pigs. Arch. Biochem. 18: 271-277, 1948.

50 For information about gossypol and digestive enzymes, see: Conkerton, E. J., and V. L. Frampton: Reaction of gossypol with free epsilon-amino groups of lysine in proteins. Arch. Biochem. Biophy. 1959; 81:130-4; Cater, C. M., and C. M. Lyman. Reactions of Gossypol with amino acids and other amino compounds. J. Amer. Oil. Chem. Soc. 1969; 46:649-653; Lyman, C. M., Baliga, B. P. and M. W. Slay. Reactions of Proteins with Gossypol. Archives of Biochemistry and Biophysics. 1959; 84:486-497.

51 Withers, W. A., and Carruth, F. E., Gossypol, The toxic substance in cottonseed meal. J. Agric. Research, 1915; 5(7): 261-283.

52 Morgan, S., Stair, E. L., Martin, T., Edwards, W. C., and G. L. Morgan. (1988) Clinical, clinicopathologic, pathologic, and toxicologic alterations associated with gossypol toxicosis in feeder lambs. American Journal of Veterinary Research. 49(4): 493-499.

53 Ferguson, T.L., Wales, J.H., Sinnhuber, R. O. and D. J. Lee. (1976) Cholesterol Levels, Atherosclerosis and Liver morphology

in rabbits fed cyclopropenoid fatty acids. <u>Food Cosmetology and Toxicology</u>. 14:15-18.

54 I discuss the problem of cottonseed and high cholesterol in chapter 2 and again in Appendix A, where I look at how other cottonseed toxins, cyclopropenoid fatty acids (CPFA's), cause high cholesterol in the blood.

55 Scientists should also research whether cottonseed toxins cause osteoporosis. I was not able to conduct the bone studies necessary to determine whether the animals in my experiment had developed osteoporosis, but the same mechanisms may be involved. Bones, like other parts of the body, are constantly evolving and changing, being broken down and rebuilt. Building bone requires the body to make a protein matrix. The body then places calcium on the bones. If the body cannot make a proper protein matrix, or if the protein matrix does not place the calcium on it properly, then the bones will not be as strong. The result will be weaker bones.

56 Nordenskjold, M. and B. Lambert. (1984) Gossypol induces DNA strand breaks in human fibroblasts and sister chromatid exchanges in human lymphocytes in vitro. <u>Journal of Medical Genetics</u>, 21, 129-132

57 O'Roak, B. J., Vives, L. Girirajan, S., Karakoc, E., Krumm, N., Coe, B. P., Levy, R., Ko, A., Lee, C., Smith, J. D., Turner, E. H., Stanaway, I. B., Vernot, B., Malig, M., Baker, C., Reilly, B., Akey, J. M., Borenstein, E., Rieder, M. J., Nickerson, D. A., Bernier, R., Shendure, J., Eichler, E. E., Sporadic autism exomes reveal a highly interconnected protein network of de novo mutations. <u>Nature</u>. 2012, Apr. 4; 485(7397):246-50

Chapter 8:

58 Morgan, S., Stair, E. L., Martin, T., Edwards, W. C., and G. L. Morgan. (1988) Clinical, clinicopathologic, pathologic, and

toxicologic alterations associated with gossypol toxicosis in feeder lambs. American Journal of Veterinary Research. 49(4): 493-499.

59 Bruce Semon and Lori Kornblum, *Feast* Without *Yeast: 4 Stages to Better Health* (1999); Bruce Semon and Lori Kornblum, *An Extraordinary Power to Heal* (2003); Lori Kornblum and Bruce Semon, *Extraordinary Foods for the Everyday Kitchen* (2003)

60 Semon, Bruce. Dietary intake of cottonseed toxins is hypothesized to be a partial cause of Alzheimer's disorder. (2012) *Medical Hypotheses*. 78: 293-298.

61 Morgan, S., Stair, E. L., Martin, T., Edwards, W. C., and G. L. Morgan. (1988) Clinical, clinicopathologic, pathologic, and toxicologic alterations associated with gossypol toxicosis in feeder lambs. American Journal of Veterinary Research. 49(4): 493-499

Appendix A:

62 Withers, W. A., and Carruth, F. E., (1915) Gossypol, The toxic substance in cottonseed meal. J. Agric. Research,. 5(7): 261-283.

63 Withers and, W. A., and F. E. Carruth.(1918) Gossypol, The toxic substance in cottonseed meal. J. Agric. Research, 12:83-101.

64 Clark, E. P. (1927) Studies on Gossypol. I. The preparation, purification, and some of the properties of gossypol, the toxic principle of cottonseed. J. Biol Chem. 75:725-739.

65 Harms, W. S., and K. T. Holley. (1951) Hypoprothrombinemia Induced by Gossypol. Proc. Soc. For Experimental Biology and Medicine. 77:297-299.

66 Hale, F. and C. M. Lyman. (1957) Effect of protein level in the rations on gossypol tolerance in growing-fattening pigs. J. Anim. Sci. 16:364.

67 Eagle, E., Castillon, L. E., Hall, C. M., and C. H. Boatner. (1948) Acute Oral Toxicity of Gossypol and Cottonseed pigment Glands for Rats, Mice, Rabbits, and Guinea Pigs. Arch. Biochem. 18: 271-277.

68 Boatner, C. H., Altschul, A. M., Irving, G., W., Jr., Pollard, E. F., and Schaeffer, H. C.,. (1948) The nutritive value of cottonseed for chicks as affected by methods of processing and content of pigment glands. Poultry Science. 27:315-328.

69 Albrecht, J. E., Clawson, A. J., Ulberg, L. C. and F. H. Smith. (1968) Effect of High Gossypol Cottonseed Meal on the Electrocardiogram of Swine. J. Anim. Sci. 27:976-980.

70 Morgan, S., Stair, E. L., Martin, T., Edwards, W. C., and G. L. Morgan. (1988) Clinical, clinicopathologic, pathologic, and toxicologic alterations associated with gossypol toxicosis in feeder lambs. American Journal of Veterinary Research. 49(4): 493-499.

71 Ambrose, A. M., and D. J. Robbins. (1951) Studies on the Chronic oral toxicity of cottonseed meal and cottonseed pigment glands. Journal of Nutrition. 43:357-70.

72 Medrano, F. J. and J. M. Andreu. (1986) Binding of gossypol to purified tubulin and inhibition of its assembly into microtubules. Eur. J. Biochem. 158(1):63-9.

73 I have no exact reference for this. I read a number of journal articles on this subject when I was at the National Cancer Institute and this possibility of permanent male infertility was mentioned but I do not have the exact citation.

74 Murthy, S. N., Wilson, H. H., Lukas, T. J., Kuret, J., Lorand, L. (1998) Cross-linking sites of the human tau protein, probed by reactions with human transglutaminase. J. Neurochem. 71(6):2607-14.

75 Abou-Donia, M. B. (1976) Physiological effects and metabolism of gossypol. Residue Rev. 61:125-60.

76 Conkerton, E. J., and V. L. Frampton: (1959) Reaction of gossypol with free epsilon-amino groups of lysine in proteins. Arch. Biochem. Biophysics. 81:130-4.

77 Conkerton, E. J., and V. L. Frampton: (1959) Reaction of gossypol with free epsilon-amino groups of lysine in proteins. Arch. Biochem. Biophysics. 81:130-4.

78 Cater, C. M., and C. M. Lyman. (1969) Reactions of Gossypol with amino acids and other amino compounds. J. Amer. Oil. Chem. Soc. 46:649-653.

79 Lyman, C. M., Baliga, B. P. and M. W. Slay. Reactions of Proteins with Gossypol. Archives of Biochemistry and Biophysics. 1959; 84:486-497.

80 Smith, F.H., and A. J. Clawson. (1965) Effect of Diet on Accumulation of Gossypol in the Organs of Swine. Journal of Nutrition. 87: 317-321.

81 Sharma, M. P., Smith, F. H. and A. J. Clawson. (1966) Effects of Levels of Protein and Gossypol, and Length of Feeding Period on the Accumulation of Gossypol in Tissues of Swine. Journal of Nutrition, 88:434-438.

82 Nordenskjold, M. and B. Lambert. (1984) Gossypol induces DNA strand breaks in human fibroblasts and sister chromatid exchanges in human lymphocytes in vitro. Journal of Medical Genetics, 21, 129-132

83 O'Roak, B. J., Vives, L. Girirajan, S., Karakoc, E., Krumm, N., Coe, B. P., Levy, R., Ko, A., Lee, C., Smith, J. D., Turner, E. H., Stanaway, I. B., Vernot, B., Malig, M., Baker, C., Reilly, B., Akey,

J. M., Borenstein, E., Rieder, M. J., Nickerson, D. A., Bernier, R., Shendure, J., Eichler, E. E., Sporadic autism exomes reveal a highly interconnected protein network of de novo mutations. Nature. 2012, Apr. 4; 485(7397):246-50

84 Shenstone, F. S. and J. R. Vickery. (1959). Substances in plants of the order Malvales causing pink whites in stored eggs. Poultry Science. 38:1055-1070.

85 Tennent, D. M., Zanetti, M. E., Siegel, H., Kuron, G. W and Ott, W. H. (1959). The influence of selected vegetable fats on plasma lipid concentrations and aortic atheromatosis in cholesterol-fed and diethylstilbestrol-implanted cockerels. J. Nutrition. 69, 283-88.

86 Tennent, D. M., Zanetti, M. E., Siegel, H., Kuron, G. W and Ott, W. H. (1959). The influence of selected vegetable fats on plasma lipid concentrations and aortic atheromatosis in cholesterol-fed and diethylstilbestrol-implanted cockerels. J. Nutrition. 69, 283-88.

87 Shenstone, F. S. and J. R. Vickery. (1961) Occurrence of Cyclo-Propene Acids in Some plants of the Order Malvales. Nature. 190:168-169.

88 Goodnight, K. C., Jr. and A. R. Kemmerer. (1967) Influence of Cyclopropenoid Fatty Acids on the Cholesterol Metabolism of Cockerels. Journal of Nutrition. 91:174-178.

89 Ferguson, T.L., Wales, J.H., Sinnhuber, R. O. and D. J. Lee. (1976) Cholesterol Levels, Atherosclerosis and Liver morphology in rabbits fed cyclopropenoid fatty acids. Food Cosmetology and Toxicology. 14:15-18.

90 Matlock, J. P., and J. E. Nixon. (1986). Impaired Clearance, Elimination, and Metabolism of Plasma Cholesterol Esters Associated with Hypercholesteremia in Mice Fed Cyclopropenoid Fatty Acids. Toxicology and Applied Pharmacology. 84:3-11.

91 Reiser, R., and Raju, P. K. (1964). The inhibition of saturated fatty acid dehydrogenation by dietary fat containing sterculic and malvalic acids. Biochem. Biophys. Res. Commun. 17:8-11.

92 Johnson, A. R., Person, J. A. Shenstone, F. S. and Fogerty, A. C. (1967). Inhibition of the desaturation of stearic to oleic acid by cylopropene fatty acid. Nature (London) 214:1244-1245.

93 Matlock, J. P., and J. E. Nixon. (1986). Impaired Clearance, Elimination, and Metabolism of Plasma Cholesterol Esters Associated with Hypercholesteremia in Mice Fed Cyclopropenoid Fatty Acids. Toxicology and Applied Pharmacology. 84:3-11.

94 Ferguson, T.L., Wales, J.H., Sinnhuber, R. O. and D. J. Lee. (1976) Cholesterol Levels, Atherosclerosis and Liver morphology in rabbits fed cyclopropenoid fatty acids. Food Cosmetology and Toxicology. 14:15-18.

95 Ayres, J. L., Lee, D. J., Wales, J. H. and Sinnhuber, R. O., Aflatoxin structure and hepatocarcinogenicity in rainbow trout (salm gairdneri). J. National. Cancer Inst. 46:561, 1971.

96 Eisele, T. A., Loveland, P. M., Kruk, D. L., Meyers, T. R., Sinnhuber, R. O. and J. E. Nixon. (1982) Effect of cyclopropenoid fatty acids on the hepatic microsomal mixed-function-oxidase system and aflatoxin metabolism in rabbits. Food and Chemical Toxicology. 20:407-412.

97 Roehm, J. N., Lee, D. J. and R. O. Sinnhuber, and S. D. Polityka. (1971). Deposition of Cyclopropenoids in the Tissue Lipids of Rainbow Trout Fed Methyl Sterculate. Lipids. 6(6): 426-430.

98 Roehm, J. N., Lee, D. J. and R. O. Sinnhuber, and S. D. Polityka. (1971). Deposition of Cyclopropenoids in the Tissue Lipids of Rainbow Trout Fed Methyl Sterculate. Lipids. 6(6): 426-430.

99 Hawkins, G.E., Cummins, K. A., Silverio, M. and J. J. Jilek. (1985). Physiological Effects of Whole Cottonseed in the Diet of Lactating Dairy Cows. J. Dairy Science. 68:2608-2614.

Appendix C:

100 Howard, J. W. and T. Fazio. (1969) A review of Polycyclic Aromatic Hydrocarbons in Foods. Agricultural and Food Chemistry, v. 17(3): 527-531.

Lijinsky, W., and P. Shubik. (1964) Benzo(a)pyrene and other Polynuclear Hydrocarbons in Charcoal-Broiled Meat. Science 145: 53-55.

Lijinsky, W. and A. E. Ross. (1967) Production of carcinogenic polynuclear hydrocarbons in the cooking of food. Food and Cosmet. Toxicol. 5, 343.

101 Bailey, E., J., and N. Dungal. (1958) Polycyclic Hydrocarbons in Icelandic Smoked Food. British Journal of Cancer. 12: 348-350.

Appendix D:

102 *farm.ewg.org/progdetail.php?fips=00000&progcode=cotton, referenced on 02/03/2013*

103 *www.alz.org › Alzheimer's Disease referenced on 02/03/2013*

104 www.cdc.gov/nccdphp/publications/aag/dhdsp.htm, *referenced on 02/03/2013*

105 www.cottoninc.com/fiber/AgriculturalDisciplines/Cottonseed/ *referenced on 02/03/2013*

www.ingramcontent.com/pod-product-compliance
Lightning Source LLC
Chambersburg PA
CBHW070758290326
41931CB00011BA/2060